Emotional Vertigo

There are few people who have never experienced vertigo, and in many instances the symptom has a psychic rather than a physical cause. In this book, Danielle Quinodoz gives an account of various forms of emotional vertigo, drawing on both Freudian and Kleinian theory to support her definition of the symptom as an expression of anxiety connected with movements in space and time.

Through numerous clinical examples the author describes different types of vertigo which appear to express different anxieties. Among these are fusion-related vertigo, vertigo related to being dropped, vertigo due to attraction to the void and competition-related vertigo, this latter appearing in an oedipal context. Through this description of Danielle Quinodoz' clinical work we gain insight into the vicissitudes in object relationships and the role of the analyst in making the patient aware of the psychological cause of the symptom. The analysand experiences the transformation of sensation into representation and is able to understand vertigo as a reflection of earliest relationships, rather than as an alien and incomprehensible symptom.

Danielle Quinodoz goes on to make the link between anxiety and pleasure by examining why we are attracted to sports in which we confront the void or vertiginous slopes. Patients often experience vertigo as a split-off part of their ego, enjoying risk-taking as if on a quest to push back the boundaries of life and time. Thus, Quinodoz argues, vertigo is inexorably linked with equilibrium, suspended as it is in a paradoxical position between anxiety and pleasure.

Emotional Vertigo offers a unique insight into object relationships and its resonance in bodily symptoms.

Danielle Quinodoz is a psychoanalyst in private practice in Geneva. She is also a training psychoanalyst of the Swiss Psychoanalytic Society and consultant at the Department of Psychiatry, University of Geneva.

ALSO IN THIS SERIES

NEW LIBRARY OF PSYCHOANALYSIS

General editor: Elizabeth Bott Spillius

Emotional Vertigo

Between Anxiety and Pleasure

DANIELLE QUINODOZ

Foreword by Alain Gibeault
Translated by Arnold Pomerans

First published as *Le Vertige entre angoisse et plaisir*,
Presses Universitaires de France, 1994

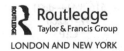

Routledge
Taylor & Francis Group

LONDON AND NEW YORK

First published as *Le Vertige entre angoisse et plaisir* in 1994
by Presses Universitaires de France, Paris

First published in English in 1997
by Routledge
4 Park Square, Milton Park, Abingdon, Oxon OX14 4RN

Simultaneously published in USA and Canada
by Routledge
605 Third Avenue, New York, NY 10017

Routledge is an imprint of the Taylor & Francis Group, an informa business

Translation © Arnold Pomerans

Typeset in Bembo by M Rules

British Library Cataloguing in Publication Data

A catalogue record for this book is available from the British Library

Library of Congress Cataloging in Publication Data

Quinodoz, Danielle
[Vertige, entre angoisse et plaisir. English]
Emotional vertigo, between anxiety and pleasure / Danielle Quinodoz ;
with a preface by Alain Gibeault ; translated by Arnold Pomerans.
p. cm. — (New library of psychoanalysis ; 28)
Includes bibliographical references and indexes.
1. Vertigo—Psychological aspects. 2. Psychoanalysis.
3. Object relations (Psychoanalysis) 4. Medicine, Psychosomatic.
5. Anxiety. 6. Pleasure. I. Title. II. Series.
RB150.V4Q5613 1997
616.8'41—dc21
97-12260
CIP

ISBN 978-0-415-14836-8 (pbk)
ISBN 978-0-415-14835-1 (hbk)

Contents

Foreword

In this fascinating book, Danielle Quinodoz suggests a way of researching and understanding vertigo, namely treating it as a factor of prototypical importance in the organization of the psyche and of its object relations. While other authors may have referred to the subject, this is the first time that vertigo and its corollary, anxiety related to the void and to falling, have been treated as part of a much wider problematic.

The author rightly recalls that Freud discussed vertigo at the very beginning of his work: at the time, he considered vertigo as an important symptom of anxiety neurosis, that is, as an example of failure to elaborate a somatic tension psychically; in addition, he also thought that it could serve as a psychic representation, especially in the case of hysterical patients.

Seen in that light, vertigo is part of a wider problematic of somatization, and can assume different functions according to whether the ego excludes or includes the body and the object. The Freudian distinction between actual neurosis and psychoneurosis which underlies the different meanings and functions of vertigo is not, however, as clear as one might think because, even in hysteria, the somatic symptom is part of the wider issue of affect prevailing over representation, and action over thinking. At times, vertigo may therefore seem a veritable form of acting out in the body intended to avoid destructive acting out with respect to the object, and to the maternal object in particular; but it also becomes an appeal during analysis to transform action into *representation* and to integrate messages from the body and from objects on the psychic plane.

This is why Danielle Quinodoz is right to consider vertigo an 'alarm system' which draws attention to faults in the containing function of the object, but which also triggers off attempts to integrate *incompatible sensations* into *representations increasingly reorganized according to the secondary process.* In these circumstances, the description of different forms of vertigo is particularly instructive, because it brings out the importance of different mediations involving the transition from sensation to representation, from passivity to activity, and from pre-oedipal forms to oedipal forms of vertigo. These mediations bear witness to a process of symbolization corresponding to an act of transformation, to a change from non-sense to sense, which Freud likened to a leap from quantity to quality.

Seen in that light, vertigo brings out the paradoxical and privileged position of the body which, while being part of external reality, is also the source of psychic reality. This presupposes that psychic work is an appropriation of the erogenous body, that is, a transformation of a body experienced as external to the self into an internal body. Danielle Quinodoz gives numerous clinical examples of the work involved in the 'decondensation' of vertigo during therapy: this is not a linear development, reflecting an inevitable transition from one form to another, but a process that brings the analyst face to face with the conflictual nature of various types of vertigo – so many modes of cathexis in conflict with one another.

Viewed from that angle, vertigo is inherent in the experience of satisfaction, because it appears the moment the *illusion* of absolute satisfaction comes up against the disillusionment of irremediable object-loss. This fact was stressed by Ferenczi in his own way when he attributed vertigo to a *sudden* change of physical and psychic attitude at the end of the session, during the possibly violent transition from the pleasure principle to the reality principle. Now, when dealing with that experience, which might entail splitting of the ego and depersonalization, we might follow Milner (1952) and Winnicott (1951) in postulating a transitional space and a transitional time that helps to maintain, however briefly, the sphere of illusion in a flow that is opposite in direction but not in essence to that of disillusionment.

This is why our understanding of vertigo, as a symptom reflecting the vacillation of space, must be linked to the psyche's experience of time. As Danielle Quinodoz stressed in connection with the dialectical relationship between vertigo and equilibrium, it involves 'playing with space and time', moving between 'change and constancy', between 'the instantaneous, and time as duration'. Hence, though vertigo is bound up with the experience of the void, we must not forget that the void is not primary but secondary, because the object is cathected in accordance with affects and rhythms, before being apprehended and lost. It is a well-known fact that the void corresponds less to a primary reality than to a phantasy, namely that of providing protection against the irruption of drives and of the object, which challenge narcissistic continuity.

Only by thus introducing the dimension of time can we transcend the absolute opposition between Being and Nothingness, to which the experience of vertigo, which engulfs the subject, takes us back. Once object-loss is felt to be definite, fixity replaces constancy, mobility replaces movement and the juxtaposition of opposites replaces contradiction. It is this temptation of dead time, which corresponds to the coexistence of two apparently incompatible attitudes, that Danielle Quinodoz has described so strikingly as the source of pathologial vertigo and of our sense of infinity. In this connection, one cannot help linking vertigo to the experience of the 'uncanny' which Freud (1919) has shown to spring from the coincidence of phantasized and external reality, and which takes us to the frontiers of the ego. It is impossible to go beyond dead time without a process of temporalization introducing a delay, a waiting period, a gap between narcissistic cathexis (I am the breast) and object cathexis (I have it, that is, I am not it) cf. Freud 1914). In that way the psychic topic is organized; it presupposes the non-simultaneity of perception (succession) and memory (constancy). The 'nihilating' effect (Sartre 1966: 804) of vertigo cannot be surmounted unless 'consciousness arises instead of a memory trace' and not at the same time (Freud 1920: 25).

Pascal (1648) observed that 'the space occupied by the void lies halfway between matter and nothingness'. That is one way of underlining the importance of negative psychic work, which can certainly engender experiences of pathological vertigo, but can also encourage the construction of psychic space and time, enabling us to discover, not the opposition of, but the difference between, Being and Nothingness. Hence we must suppose that this 'potential space' is also an 'intermediate area of experience' (Winnicott 1971), mediating relations between the internal and the external world: a third space thus constituting the crucible or matrix of all symbolization by the fusion of the ego with the non-ego which alone allows us to differentiate between them, and to take shelter from vertiginous collapse.

The construction of that dimension, which has enabled Danielle Quinodoz to reconcile extremes, can then give rise to 'games' involving different forms of vertigo and facilitating a transition from anxiety to pleasure. This clearly calls for emotional work in correlation with the integration of the *receptivity* that is so indispensable to human experience, and in that sense constitutes a major investment in all analytic treatments. One of the merits of this book is that it invites us to reflect, with the help of a wide range of clinical examples, on the essential role vertigo plays in the psyche, and to muse with the author about the many transformations of that experience in the most varied facets of the pleasure principle inherent in psychic life.

Alain Gibeault

References

Freud, S. (1914) 'On Narcissism: an Introduction', SE 14: 67–105.
—— (1919) *The 'Uncanny'*, SE 17: 218–256.
—— (1920) *Beyond the Pleasure Principle*, SE 18: 1–64.
Milner, M. (1952) 'Aspects of symbolism in comprehension of the not-self', in *International Journal of Psycho-Analysis*, 33: 181–195.
Pascal, B. (1648) *Récit de la grande expérience de l'équilibre des liqueurs*, Paris: Charles Savram, quoted in D. Anzieu, 'Naissance du concept de vide chez Pascal, *Nouvelle Revue de psychanalyse*, 1975, 11: 195–203.
Sartre, J.-P. (1966) *Being and Nothingness*, New York: Washington Square Press.
Winnicott, D.W. (1951) 'Transitional objects and transitional phenomena', in *Through Paediatrics to Psycho-Analysis*, London: Hogarth, pp. 229–242.
—— (1971) *Playing and Reality*, Harmondsworth: Penguin.

1

What is vertigo?

I became interested in vertigo a long time ago – when Luc first came to consult me: he complained of vertigo and asked for psychoanalysis. His vertigo hampered him considerably, not only in his social and leisure activities, but also in his professional life. He had previously seen a number of physicians who had failed to detect a somatic cause. In the end, his family doctor, who had found Luc in perfect health, had advised him to consult a psychoanalyst. Luc had hesitated; he had first tried self-analysis, reading Freud and using introspection, but his vertigo had become more acute. He had then decided to see a psychoanalyst: he felt vaguely that his vertigo might be connected with his way of relating to people important to him; he also sensed that, if relationship problems were really involved, communication with the analyst would help him to get to the bottom of them. Actually, though he had not thought it through, Luc felt vaguely that he was in danger of repeating his relationship problems in the transference, and hoped that the analyst might help him to bring these problems into the open and to change them.

Luc simply said that he had vertigo. But what kind of vertigo? What was its precise nature? At first he mentioned his insurmountable fear of falling out of a cable-car; but that fear quickly turned out to be no more than a gateway to a very complex world: the world of vertigo.

Definitions

The various meanings of the word 'vertigo'

In current French, the word *vertige* can refer to a variety of symptoms. To begin with, there is a difference between *vertige* – vertigo – and *vertiges* – giddy spells. If you say that you suffer from the first, you are indicating that

1

you have a fear of heights or suffer from mountain sickness; in the second case you convey the fact that you tend to feel dizzy and may be physically ill. However, with these two meanings the ambiguities only begin, not only in the somatic but also in the psychic realm.

In fact, the expression *I have vertigo* can be used to express a physical sensation (for example, 'I feel the room is starting to spin'), but it can also reflect a feeling of disquiet or anxiety about a psychologically daunting situation (for example, 'The immensity of the task before me makes me feel giddy'), in which case the physical sensation of vertigo betrays a particular form of psychic or emotional insecurity.

Even when people say 'I feel giddy' to describe their physical sensations, we realize that they might be referring to a number of quite distinct experiences. What, then, do we mean by vertigo?

The word *vertigo* is derived from the Latin *vertere*, to turn; it reflects the mistaken impression that our surroundings revolve round us, but also the opposite false impression, that it is we ourselves who, having lost our balance, keep spinning involuntarily. Professor Rudolf Häusler, an oto-neurologist who is particularly interested in vertigo, provided this definition during his course of lectures at the Geneva faculty of medicine (1989): 'Vertigo reflects a mistaken sensation of the body's movement in space, or of the movement of space with respect to the body. It can give rise to a feeling of turning, reeling, or of the imminent danger of falling.'

He also distinguishes between vertigo (*vertige*), dizziness (*malaise*), and loss of balance (*déséquilibre*), three terms that are often confused in modern French. In the *Journal: Questions et Réponses*, he proffered the following explanations:

'*Vertige*' is derived from vertigo, which means whirling. The term therefore applies above all to rotatory feelings but can also describe the sensation of rolling, of pitching and tossing, or of an imminent fall. In short, it therefore refers to a disturbance of the perception of space combined with an illusion of movement.

'*Malaise*' generally refers to an acute condition coupled to a sense of weakness, of being empty-headed, of having lost one's physical and mental powers, and often of feeling faint ('presyncopal state'). *Malaise* includes a whole range of neuro-vegetative manifestations such as cold sweats, nausea, vomiting, abdominal cramps, irregular pulse, and drop in blood pressure. It can even include rotatory vertiginous sensations.

'*Déséquilibre*' refers to disturbances of the postural sense, especially while one is stationary before or during a walk . . .

In modern usage, the terms '*vertige*', '*malaise*' and '*déséquilibre*', inasmuch as they refer to medical complaints, tend to overlap. They may describe not only the sensations listed above, but also such purely psychic

2

disturbances as phobias (fear of heights = void-related vertigo, agora-phobia) and depressive states (vertigo felt in the face of an insurmountable problem, the condition manifesting itself before a difficult situation).

Similarly, in respect of the clinical meaning of these terms, considered as symptoms, we find that vertigo is often accompanied by *malaise*, and also that it can cause loss of balance. In the same way, rotatory vertiginous sensations occur very often during *malaise*.

(Häusler 1985: 12)

Vertigo of emotional origin has the same symptoms as vertigo of somatic origin, and hence fits into Häusler's picture, although it is due to psychic rather than somatic causes. Nor can it be reduced to a form of vertigo elicited by particular external conditions, because, even when these conditions appear to trigger it off, they do not suffice to explain it. We must therefore try to get at the psychic mechanisms responsible for a set of symptoms that so spectacularly involve the body, and to discover what significance they have for the patients concerned.

It is obvious that, as a psychoanalyst, I should be primarily interested in vertigo of psychic origin, and that I should try to discover what psychic mechanisms might help to elicit that symptom. Even so, I shall give a brief summary of the manner in which the mechanisms of vertigo can currently be explained on the somatic level, if only to emphasize how firmly the psychic aspect is rooted in the somatic. It may be of special interest to note that the appearance of vertigo of somatic origin is connected with the difficulty of integrating the diverse data provided by different perceptual systems, and that the appearance of vertigo of psychic origin is bound up with the difficulty of integrating equally diverse psychic currents (needs, wishes, affects). Moreover, vertigo can be said to serve as an alarm signal in both cases.

Summary of the mechanisms of vertigo of somatic origin

Data provided jointly by three sensory systems

The sense of balance or of vertigo of somatic origin depends on the co-ordination of data supplied by three sensory systems: the optokinetic apparatus (optical data), the proprioceptive apparatus (which supplies data about muscles and tendons, and tells us about the position and changes in the position of the body) and the vestibular apparatus (which comprises the otolithic system and the semi-circular canals located in the internal ear, and keeps us informed about the static position of the head, about bodily movements and about gravitational pull). These three systems help us to take stock of our position and of our equilibrium in space, and to act accordingly.

Of these three, the vestibular apparatus plays the most important role. When these three systems supply coherent data, these data are integrated to provide us with a sense of balance. When one of the systems provides data that do not agree with those provided by the other two systems, then vertigo may ensue.

The disparity between the various sets of data may be of pathological origin. There may be a lesion in one of the three systems, causing that system to produce abnormal data; most often such lesions occur in the vestibular system. Thus an otolith may have been displaced and jammed; it loses its mobility and provides erroneous information about the position of the head, that information no longer corresponding to the data supplied by the other two systems, with a consequent threat of vertigo. By manipulation of the patient's head (Semon's manoeuvre), the physician can sometimes unwedge the otolith, restore its freedom of movement, help it to function normally and to provide valid information; the vertigo disappears.

Vertigo can thus serve as an alarm signal, alerting us to a possible defect in one of the three systems that combine to help us to establish our equilibrium.

The sensation of vertigo is not necessarily of pathological origin

The disparity between the data provided by the three perceptual systems need not be of pathological origin, but can be due to special external conditions with which everyone is familiar.

Suppose, for instance, that we are standing at the edge of a precipice. Our inner ear informs us that we are standing still, our proprioceptive system signals that our feet are touching the ground as usual and that our position is stable, but our optokinetic system supplies data that do not tally with those coming from the first two systems: we look at the bottom of the precipice, and see the ground a thousand yards below us. There is a discrepancy between the data: two sources make us feel the ground under our feet, but the third makes us see the ground a thousand yards below; this incoherence can give rise to a non-pathological form of vertigo of somatic origin. That explains why mountain guides sometimes tell a climber overcome by vertigo in the midst of a climb: 'Stop looking down! Look at the rock face straight in front of you!'

Now, a very interesting thing happens when the person who has vertigo at the edge of a precipice takes off with a para-glider or hang-glider: as soon as he leaves the ground his vertigo disappears. By eliminating the information that the ground is underneath his feet, he has also suppressed the disagreement between the information produced by his three sensory systems: the three systems now supply concordant data and the vertigo has vanished.

I could easily quote other, more common experiences. For instance, some people get vertigo when they read in a moving car: there is a discordance between information of vestibular origin suggesting that they are experiencing displacements, accelerations or rotations; and information from their optical system which tells them that they are looking at a stationary page of a book. If they then look at the landscape in the distance, the vertigo generally dies down. Or take the case of the person who having waltzed, say, clockwise for a long time, suddenly stops, and then feels so giddy that he is in danger of collapsing on the spot: when he stopped, his semicircular canal and otoliths, over-stimulated by the waltzing, continued to signal that he was still moving, while his optokinetic system presented him with static surroundings. The incompatibility of the data led to vertigo. Waltzers often deal with this discordance by ending their dance with a brief whirl in the opposite direction; that serves to slow down the movement of liquid in the semicircular canals, which are then able to convey the state of immobility more rapidly.

It is worth noting that these somatic mechanisms giving rise to vertigo and equilibrium do not affect everybody in the same way. Some people do not have vertigo at the edge of a precipice, some people can happily read in a moving car, and there are others who used to have vertigo at the edge of a precipice but have it no longer. Does that not suggest that some psychic component may intervene to modify the course of what is at first a purely somatic process? In fact, the person at the edge of a precipice can, by his own psychic action, correct the information received by one of his perceptual systems with the help of a partial deciphering process enabling him to restore coherence; experience and training thus play an important role and some persons subject to vertigo can, if no emotional factor is added, learn to overcome it. We also find that some people are better than others at compartmentalizing the data or at taking advantage of one system of information while pushing the rest into the background: in a car, some passengers are so absorbed by what they are reading that, to all intents and purposes, they ignore all the other information and hence do not suffer from vertigo; in short, some people have no problem in reading an exciting text in a car, but have vertigo if the text bores them.

All these facts lead us to think that a psychic component may intervene even in the case of non-pathological vertigo of somatic origin. More generally, people can learn to master physiological vertigo provided they do not also suffer from anxiety giving rise to vertigo of psychic origin.

Psychoanalysts and physicians in the face of vertigo of psychic origin

It is obvious that, as a psychoanalyst interested in the meaning of vertigo of psychic or emotional origin, I take a different view from that of Häusler and other physicians. Even so, their work and the information it provides are extremely valuable to me. Actually, in order to be able to analyse the symptoms of vertigo of psychic origin, or even the psychic components of a case of vertigo due to somatic causes, I consider it essential to obtain an expert medical opinion about the origin of the vertigo presented by patients who come to see me.

On the one hand, it is important for me to know if the specialists have been able to exclude, as far as possible, any possibility of a somatic cause; on the other hand, whenever they think that this symptom is of somatic origin, it is equally important for me to know how severe the patient's somatic condition is. In no circumstances must the diagnosis of a grave somatic illness be brushed aside, the less so as its beginnings might well have manifested themselves by that particular symptom.

On this subject, Rentchnick and Häusler mention a study of a thousand persons suffering from vertigo who were examined between 1980 and 1982 at the onto-neurological unit of the ear, nose and throat clinic attached to the Cantonal University Hospital in Geneva. Häusler states that 'in 29% of these cases it was not possible to determine the origin of the vertigo' (Rentchnick and Häusler 1985: 3097). He adds later that

> what is important is that one can almost invariably determine the origin of those cases of vertigo that were caused by a grave illness, in which an early diagnosis is vital. In fact, it is estimated that from 5% to 10% of all vertigo cases have a serious cause, for example a brain tumour or a cerebro-vascular accident that can endanger the patient's life.
>
> (*ibid*: 3098)

He concludes: 'Approximately 80% of all cases of vertigo have a spontaneous cure. This conclusion should enable the physician to reassure this group of patients '(*ibid.*: 3098).

Who turns to psychoanalysts in cases of vertigo?

The thousand cases of vertigo studied at the Geneva hospital between 1980 and 1982 are not representative of those who come to see psychoanalysts – in my own practice I have had to deal with quite different requests concerning vertigo. It is rare for vertigo to be, at least on the manifest level, the main reason for a request for psychoanalysis. However, it does happen that people ask for analysis as their last hope of being freed of a symptom that ruins their life. Generally, they have already consulted medical practitioners who failed to find a somatic cause for their vertigo. This, in particular, was the case of Luc, whose normal life was badly upset by this symptom. Luc used the general term *vertige* to describe his condition, but actually he presented all three related forms described by Häusler: vertigo, giddiness and loss of balance.

On the other hand, many analysands consulting me for reasons other than vertigo later disclosed that they suffered from this symptom; they had failed to mention it earlier either because the symptom was mild, or else because they had never thought that vertigo might have anything to do with psychoanalysis.

Moreover, I have often noticed – and many colleagues have told me that they had made the same observation – that numerous patients present isolated vertigo episodes of various forms during their analysis; this may even happen to patients who had not been subject to this complaint before to any great extent. It is therefore interesting to anyone concerned with the course of the analytic process to discover in what circumstances these episodes occurred and what their significance was.

Yet other patients consult a psychoanalyst aware that they suffer from vertigo of somatic origin, linked, for example, to Ménière's disease, and identified and treated as such by medical specialists. In no case did they expect the psychoanalyst to replace the physician, but merely to help them to live as best they could with an illness that can sometimes be very troublesome, indeed frightening. Some medical specialists will encourage them to consult a psychoanalyst, in the knowledge that medical science cannot yet eradicate the cause of their discomfort.

In psychoanalysis, we also sometimes encounter patients who seem to treat vertigo as a challenge, who play with leaps into space, and who take special pleasure in flirting with what, while threatening to give them vertigo, also provides them with thrills they need not fear. Between the pleasure afforded by heady adventures and dicing with death, there is a no man's land that may be worth exploring, however daunting the task.

I must mention yet another aspect of vertigo with which nearly all my patients have been confronted at some time during their analysis. I am referring to metaphysical vertigo caused by confronting the great existential questions: life, death, infinity, eternity, the sense of one's own being or nothingness, the feeling of emptiness. This form of vertigo is defined by the answers to such questions as 'What is the meaning of (my) life?' or 'What is the meaning of (my) death?' I sometimes wonder if the need of certain patients to find a psychic meaning for their personal history in order to improve it, is not simply one way of warding off the anxiety caused by their failure to discover a meaning in life.

Psychoanalysts and the study of vertigo

Freud kept referring to vertigo (*Schwindel*, translated as 'vertigo' by Strachey in the *Standard Edition*) throughout his writings; he considered it one of the major symptoms of anxiety neurosis. I have devoted part of Chapter 11 to the development of Freud's thought on this subject.

After Freud, to the best of my knowledge, those psychoanalysts who made a special study of the symptom of vertigo concentrated mainly on vertigo of somatic origin, thus following in the footsteps of French (1929); however, Schilder (1939) and Rycroft (1953) contended that vertigo could sometimes be linked to neurosis. Rallo (1972), using the approach of Abraham (1913), took an interest in the physical, and especially the muscular, phenomena accompanying giddiness, associating them, among other factors, with the repression of aggression. In 1990, I presented vertigo of psychic origin as a fundamental experience in the organization of the psyche, one that enables us to investigate the vicissitudes of the object relationship (D. Quinodoz, 1990d). Melanie Klein, to the best of my knowledge, did not make any explicit reference to vertigo, but dealt at great length with anxiety. That is why at the end of Chapter 11 I stress those parts of her theory of anxiety that support my view of vertigo.

Vertigo and object relationships

In my work with analysands, vertigo appeared to be an expression of anxiety manifesting itself through physical sensations connected to space and time: I was able to demonstrate that the various forms this symptom may assume during treatment reflected the vicissitudes of the analysand's relations with important persons in his inner world. These vicissitudes manifest themselves from the ability to differentiate oneself from the object[1] and then separate from it, to the emergence of what Jean-Michel Quinodoz has called the 'feeling of buoyancy' (*portance*) (J.-M. Quinodoz 1993). For me the study of vertigo is much more than the observation and description of a symptom. I believe it is a prototypical dimension of the object relationship, so much so that it can be considered to be a fundamental experience in the organization of the psyche, involving the fear of falling and a sense of inner emptiness.

It is fascinating to try to understand how vertigo, an experience of sensations that does not apparently lend itself to psychic working out – that is, as a symptom presenting itself as an accumulation of purely physical tensions – can, in the course of psychoanalysis, become organized on the psychic plane. What we have here is psychic work that makes it possible to pass from vertigo felt exclusively as a set of sensations to vertigo felt as having a function of psychic defence thanks to the binding of affects in representations. For example, the transition from the *sensation* of the void to the *feeling* of emptiness accompanied by representations demands intense psychic work. It is a call for the integration by means of representations of sensations increasingly organized according to the secondary process and that, at first, seemed impossible to link: a transition from passivity to activity, from pre-oedipal to oedipal forms of thought. It is equally interesting to gather to what great extent the analyst is forced to trust his counter-transference in order to help the analysand discover representations that will enable him to become aware of his various levels of vertigo, and to make sense of them in order to work out his conflicts by recourse to his symbolizing capacity.

Physical and psychic equilibrium; the language that touches

The medical definition of vertigo is based on the relative position of a person in his surroundings. On the somatic plane, if that position is satis-factory, the person feels stable and balanced; or rather, he is not aware of being stable as he rarely thinks about it under normal conditions; it is usu-ally not until he loses his balance that he realizes that balance did exist before. That may explain why people invent situations in games or in sports that carry them to the verge of disequilibrium, the better to enjoy the sense of being in command of their body that goes with the restoration of their balance.

A similar process occurs on the psychic plane: the ego defines itself by dif-ferentiation from its environment. According to some theories, at the start of his life, the child is not aware of being distinct from the person who looks after him; according to other theories he is aware of the presence of that object all along but in a very primitive way. We can easily imagine that when the infant feeds at the breast he does not know where the breast stops and where his own mouth begins. Indeed, he is not aware that there is a breast and a mouth, a mother and a baby. It is but gradually that a differen-tiation occurs, thanks particularly to repeated absences of the breast, which enable the baby to appreciate its former presence. This disequilibrium thus makes him aware that the breast is not his mouth, and hence that his mother is not himself. In addition to the perception of the difference between his body and his mother's, he starts to differentiate himself as a person from the person of his mother. Hence it is not merely the body which situates and defines itself by differentiation from the environment, but his entire self, including his psyche.

To me, vertigo seems an outstanding means of studying object relations, because the material produced by an analysand who talks about his vertigo, which, as Ferenczi (1914) showed, inseparably involves both the physical and the psychic dimension, enables us to analyse the vicissitudes of the object relationship in a language that evokes or recalls bodily resonances. It seemed obvious to me that the interpretations that most *touched* persons subject to vertigo were those that elicited representations with a resonance at the level of bodily sensations; I believe moreover that, in general, this is an important point in the formulation of all interpretations. These patients help us to avoid two opposite dangers that may befall us whenever we speak of the ego and its relations: the dangers of *reifying* the ego and of *rendering it abstract*; with these patients it is clear that the ego is neither a thing nor an abstraction, but 'first and foremost a body-ego' (Freud 1923b: 27).

Vertigo and the body

The clinical psychoanalyst is led to emphasize how essential it is to remember the bodily aspect if the analysand is to discover the symbolic significance of his symptom of vertigo. During analysis, the analysand will have the experience of appropriating his body-ego and come to realize that vertigo is part of a problem of somatization that assumes different meanings depending on whether his ego excludes or includes the corporeal aspect. He can, in effect, experience his vertigo as something happening outside himself, something triggered off by external events, but this experience can become positive, a source of psychic enrichment the moment he realizes that his ego, being corporeal, is involved in his vertigo.

By introducing the term *corporeal* I am trying to bring out what particularly interests me as a psychoanalyst in the study of vertigo. When I speak of the corporeal factor, I am not referring to the body as the object of rational anatomical or physiological studies, but to the internal representations of one's own body linked to unconscious bodily phantasies. The psychoanalyst lays particular emphasis on the unconscious, the phantasies of the internal world; to me that internal world is inseparable from the inner objects with which the ego entertains phantasy relationships.[2] The history of ego–object differentiation has a corporeal model: the differentiation of body and environment. We might put it that separation anxiety, which is another way of speaking of the ego–object differentiation, similarly has a corporeal expression in the anxiety of not finding the object at the appointed place and of falling into the void.

We thus catch a glimpse of the full diversity of this symptom and of the many meanings it can assume in clinical practice. In fact, this symptom has a general significance and one we encounter in numerous patients, namely that of revealing the vagaries of the object relationship and hence helping us to understand it; however, it assumes a particular meaning and a specific form with every analysand, because every analysand constructs a characteristic object relationship, depending on his originality as a subject and on that of the object. As always in psychoanalysis, we are left with conceptual perspectives applicable to all, but experienced differently by every patient at the individual clinical level. Vertigo has a particular meaning for each patient.

Differentiation: guarantee of linkage or of rupture?

A threat of rupture

The history of the relationship between the ego and its internal objects is a long story; it ends with death. Ideally, it should be the history of an ego that differentiates and separates itself gradually from its objects, not in order to abandon them or to be abandoned by them, but on the contrary to establish better communications with them. While everything is mixed up, with ego and objects confused, communication is difficult, because one expects what the other imagines one will expect; however, once differentiation has taken place, better communication is facilitated, inasmuch as one appreciates that he must 'open himself' to the other if he is to be understood, which leads him to define himself, to make himself increasingly clear. In that case, the links created between the ego and the objects become increasingly rich, and entail the ever-growing creation of new links joining up, in an increasingly dense network, with previous links.

Now, it is far from obvious that a person's history must unfold in that particular direction. When an analysand differentiates himself from persons important to him, anxiety may ensue: the separation, instead of entailing new links, may then lead to rupture. Indeed, the recognition of the differences between, and the limits of, the ego and the object imply giving up control of the object – that is, abandoning the wish to force it into similitude – and instead to take an interest in the disclosure of its distinctiveness and the communications to which it can give rise. That presupposes a mode of relationship based on freedom and trust. Now, the object left free was left free precisely not to respond to the subject's desire for communication. The intention of defining oneself in all one's particularity may pose the threat of eliciting a rejection by objects felt to be capable of refusing to accept the difference.

Is the risk worth taking?

This threat proves a source of anxiety some patients find hard to accept:

> Delimiting oneself from the object, that is, accepting the space of separation between ego and object, implies that the analysand values the relationship he has established with a free object so highly that he is prepared to lose the object rather than keep it by force, as he would in a fusion-based relationship.
>
> (D. Quinodoz 1989c: 1648)

For some analysands it is much too frightening to take the risk of losing the object which they delude themselves into thinking they can preserve by fusion; they cannot decide to give up that relative security and take a leap into what they fear is the void.

However, those patients who are most afraid of discovering this space of separation are just the ones who need it most. The breaking down of the boundaries between the ego and the object causes a narcissistic haemorrhage of the ego, often felt as an insupportable loss of the sense of existence; Alain Gibeault (1989) has stressed that these narcissistic patients have a need to bump against the limits of the object in order to stop that haemorrhage and to discover their own limits, but that, at the same time, they experience extreme anxiety at being torn apart as they perceive the limits against which they nevertheless persist in flinging themselves.

Their anxiety is all the greater because they find it hard to imagine any other mode of relationship than the fusional; they can only see two possibilities, one as unsatisfactory as the other: the illusion of communication in fusion, and the relational void outside the fusion. That is why they often choose to regress to fusion the moment they detect differences in thought and feelings between their analyst and themselves.

Universality of the symptoms of vertigo; universality of the experiences of falling and absence

Nearly everyone has had vertigo

I have been surprised to find that, in general, the term vertigo leaves no one indifferent. It seems to me that it is very rare to meet anyone who can say that he has never had it, for instance as a child in the form of play, when an adult pretended to drop him. Now the memory of an episode of vertigo is always impressive; vertigo almost invariably takes us by surprise and is experienced by us in the incommunicable seclusion of bodily experience. One analysand told me: 'What I experienced that day is something I can describe, but no one except myself could feel what I experienced.'

Everybody has had the personal experience of deciding whether or not to let go of their support; everybody has had the experience of falling

The universal character of the vertigo experience is interesting because, as always, normal experiences tend to go unobserved; it is when something goes wrong that we become aware of what we usually take for granted. In the child's normal development, which generally leads it to let go of its supports or its props bit by bit, and to adapt itself increasingly to the exigencies of the environment until it is able to walk unaided, the child must often wonder if it can let go of a particular support; if it can recover its support; and if it can leave a space between itself and the support. If the answers are positive, everything goes smoothly. But the child's assessment may be wrong and he then has the experience of falling, something that has happened to all of us.

That experience can, however, be very fruitful if the child makes the right use of it; it can even be considered indispensable in the child's learning to assess its adjustment to the environment correctly. However, the fall may also be remembered as a scenario to be avoided, as a frightening failure in the child's adjustment to the object. That scenario is enacted in vertigo. Now such games as the one played by an uncle who pretends to drop a child but catches it again in the air, a game described by Freud as extraordinarily attractive to children (1900a: 271), enable us precisely to play with the experience of letting go of our support without falling into the void. This is one way of playing with what might give us vertigo.

However, there may be failures as well as pleasant games. The failures are sometimes due to the object, but also to the subject, to their relationship and the phantasies the subject projects into the object: for example, though the object is objectively present, the ego may project terrifying phantasies into it and fail to recognize it, so much so that the object is felt to be absent at the level of internal reality. The fall or the absence of the object may then, at worst, give rise to anxiety and remain an experience of psychic vertigo as the expression of anxiety; at best they may linger on as the awareness that a fall as a 'psychic fall' is possible and that perhaps the feeling of falling into the void could occur. Every one of us knows that the normal development of children learning to walk by themselves involves the experience of falling down and that the normal experience of learning to be oneself, as distinct from others, involves the feeling of falling into a void.

This shows how inseparable corporeal experience is from psychic experience. Does the child play in order to discover the position of his body with respect to a support? In that case we should have a mainly physical experience. Does the child play in order to differentiate himself from the person who looks after him, or does he let go of her, having just enough fear of being abandoned to appreciate the assurance of not having been deserted? In that case we should have a mainly psychic experience. What we have here in fact is the general scenario of vertigo: will the object be where I expect it to be, or am I going to fall into the void? It is no longer a matter of adjusting the body to the environment or of adjusting the ego to the personality of the other; what we have here is a total adjustment of the bodily ego to the internal objects, the bodily ego expressing that inseparable unity of the ego whose psychic dimension is rooted in the bodily dimension and revealed by it.

13

André Green's use of the term 'blanche'

In their *L'Enfant de ça*, Donnet and Green mention *psychose blanche* in connection with a patient who had giddy spells among other symptoms
(Donnet and Green 1973: 58). Going on to define this use of the term
'blanche' ('whitey'), André Green adds several clarifications that have a
bearing on sensations of empty space and on vertigo:

> 'blanche' in the sense in which I use it is derived from the English *blank*,
> which refers to an unoccupied space (left, for example, for a signature at
> the bottom of a form, or for the figures on a blank cheque . . .). The
> Anglo-Saxon term comes from the French *blanc*, which refers to a
> colour . . . We are thus up against a semantic bifurcation: the colour, *albus*
> in Latin vs. empty space, the *blank* of the Anglo-Saxons.
>
> (Green 1983: 156)

The association of these two meanings of *blanc* agrees well with the symptom of vertigo. In fact, the corporeal sensation of vertigo is intrusive and fills
the entire space left by the absence of ideas and of symbolism. For example,
the analysand does not have the least idea which internal object it is that
drops him or what affect he feels in his object relationship, although he suffers from it (*blank*); at the same time, however, his conscious space is
completely invaded by the sensation of vertigo (*white colour*) which masks the
lack (void) of ideas. Hence, with the particular manifestation of anxiety we
refer to as vertigo, we are led back, on the one hand, to the importance of
the disappearance of the mediation provided by representation, and, on the
other hand, to the self-expulsion of the ego, with the paradoxical quasi-
simultaneity of the internal void trying to oppose the intrusive motion
which has been filling the void; we also discover that the instinctive motion
has bodily roots.

A clinical example: a request for analysis in a case of vertigo

Theoretical considerations rooted in clinical experience

The work done in psychoanalysis takes place on the psychic level, but the
psyche is rooted in the corporeal, and the analysis of vertigo seems to me an
outstanding way of getting at that root. When we speak of man's corporeal
aspect we are referring to what is unique in what every person senses, feels
and thinks. That means that our reflections spring from the solitude of our
own experience, even when we subject it to the most wide-ranging study:
it is from my relationship with my patients that my ideas about vertigo have
taken shape, and that is why I have chosen to illustrate this book with

personal cases culled from my clinical practice and especially from my psychoanalytic treatment of Luc.

In Luc's case, the changes in the forms and meanings of the symptom of vertigo ran like a red thread through his analysis. Professional ethics prevent me from discussing Luc's case in detail, or those objects in his history whom I represented for him in the transference, with all the instinctual and conflictual aspects that implies. I shall merely provide a few clinical vignettes strictly linked to his vertigo. As a result, even if the reflections and phantasies I mention are authentic, no one will be able to recognize himself as the Luc of these pages; by contrast each one of us may perhaps see himself in some twist or another of the clinical accounts that follow.

Splitting: vertigo spares the person as a whole

Clearly, not all analysands afflicted with general anxiety, separation anxiety or castration anxiety present the symptom of vertigo. I have noticed that many patients who suffer from vertigo as a manifestation of anxiety have attained a good level of personal development as a whole; however, through their symptom, they present a regressive part of their ego, contrasting with their general level of development. Vertigo allows some sort of localization of anxiety, and this has the advantage of protecting the person as a whole, at least to some extent. I say *to some extent* because we know from experience that an encapsulated or split-off emotional state cannot leave the person as a whole untouched; the same thing happens on the somatic plane: a local inflammation hampers the whole of our activity, even if it does so to a lesser extent than a widespread inflammation. Vertigo seems to me most often a manifestation of anxiety felt and expressed in a *split-off* part of the patient's ego, in the sense Freud uses that term in his *Outline of Psychoanalysis* (1940a [1938]). In that work, Freud points out that it is common to find two simultaneous, contrary and independent attitudes in patients, no matter if their condition is more psychotic or more neurotic.

In the first group the splitting of the ego is most often due to the perception of reality:

> Two psychical attitudes have been formed instead of a single one – one, the normal one, which takes account of reality, and another which under the influence of the instincts detaches the ego from reality. The two exist alongside of each other. The issue depends on their relative strength. If the second [attitude] is or becomes the stronger, the necessary precondition for a psychosis is present.
>
> (Freud 1940a: 202)

In the second group the process is different:

15

It is indeed a universal characteristic of neuroses that there are present in the subject's mental life, as regards some particular behaviour, two different attitudes, contrary to each other and independent of each other. In the case of neuroses, however, one of these attitudes belongs to the ego and the contrary one, which is repressed, belongs to the id.

Freud adds:

. . . it is not always easy to decide in an individual instance with which of the two possibilities one is dealing. They have, however, the following important characteristics in common. Whatever the ego does in its efforts of defence, whether it seeks to disavow a portion of the real external world or whether it seeks to reject an instinctual demand from the internal world, its success is never complete and unqualified. The outcome always lies in two contrary attitudes . . .

(*ibid.*: 204)

The various forms of vertigo reflect the simultaneous presence of two contrary attitudes (one well-adapted and well-developed and the other regressive and leading to the presentation of the symptom of vertigo), but it is not always easy to decide between them and to determine whether the regressive attitude is the result of a denial of external reality or of repression of an internal instinctual need. In any case, I believe that the more patently vertigo is a manifestation of separation anxiety, the more we are brought face to face with splitting of the ego coupled to a denial of the perceived reality; and that the more clearly vertigo is a manifestation of castration anxiety, the more we are faced with two contrary attitudes, one of which serves to repel an instinctual demand of internal origin. I have often had the impression that vertigo as a manifestation of anxiety appears in therapy, especially in grave cases, as an alarm system, when the more regressive attitude, involving the denial of reality or instinctual repression, threatens to overwhelm the patient's other attitude. I shall be returning to this point in Chapter 10.

The case of Luc: a request for psychoanalysis motivated by vertigo

During the preliminary interviews, in which Luc expressed the wish to have psychoanalytic treatment, I had the clear impression that his ego must be split. On the one hand he presented himself as a sports-loving father, well adapted to family, social and professional life, 'simply' requesting analysis in order to put a stop to his vertigo, to be able to go on ski lifts and so improve his skiing; on the other hand, he also showed me sporadic manifestations of a different kind: feelings of giddiness and breakdown accompanied by panic and loss of control of himself, thus endangering his professional and family life. These latter manifestations looked as if they came from a split-off part of Luc, but these parts were so much ignored by him that I took relatively little notice of them. Luc himself also spoke lightly of them and in a detached way, as if they were not really part of him; it was almost as if he were describing someone other than himself, someone who in any case seemed to hold little sway beside the 'well-adapted' person he presented himself to me as being.

Yet as soon as Luc lay down on the couch for his first session with me, the splitting manifested itself with full force, and I was startled to see a patient racked with anxiety, glued to the couch, agitated and trembling, breaking his silence with a stream of incoherent words: the split-off part of Luc, much more regressive than I could ever have guessed, filled the entire room. I was frightened, but then I had embarked on this analytic adventure with the whole Luc and not just with the relatively well-adapted part that had taken up nearly all our preliminary interviews.

I wondered how Luc could possibly resume normal life after he left me. But at the end of the session I had a fresh shock: Luc suddenly recovered the 'adapted' aspect of his ego, and stepped out energetically as if quite oblivious to his regressive part. I realized that he had to play his professional and social roles at the cost of radically splitting off the part of himself he did not understand. Those people around him who only knew Luc superficially must not so much as suspect the presence of his split-off part or the permanent tension caused by the fear that the split-off part might erupt into the rest of his ego, threatening to convulse the whole person.

Making differentiations within the rock of vertigo

The analysand often presents his symptom of vertigo to the analyst as a compact whole: he says 'I have vertigo' as if there were just one global form of vertigo instead of a whole range. His vertigo seems to be lacking in nuances, in differences of meaning, that is, to be devoid of a way in, of a handle by which to seize it. Now it is my firm belief that the feeling that vertigo is like a compact rock prevents it from being integrated. The compact, impenetrable rock presented by some patients made me feel as if I had vertigo myself, a little like the rocks the painter René Magritte dangles from the sky. Actually, it was at a retrospective exhibition of Magritte's work that I discovered an artistic representation of the work of differentiation (*décondensation*)[3] we perform so often in psychoanalysis and especially in cases of vertigo: the analysand first shows us his vertigo as a global whole, a rock, and nothing but a rock. Then, bit by bit, shapes stand out from that rock: there is no longer just one impenetrable vertiginous mass, but various forms of vertigo, each distinguished from the rest by different sensations and meanings. When that happens, both of us, analyst and analysand, have the feeling of gradually differentiating [*le sentiment*

17

de décondenser] this compact mass into its component parts by deploying them in space and time; we then realize that this compact vertigo is made up of a host of vertigoes which relate by combining with one another.

Similarly, if we look at Magritte's paintings, paying particular attention to a certain subject, for instance the rock, we see first of all a primitive rock which is simply a rock. But then this impenetrable rock presents us with different shapes: a fortress, a house, an interior, furniture, increasingly animated objects, a human form, a woman, and perhaps the image of the lost mother, drowned. At first this rock, painted concretely as a compact thing, was unassimilable, but as elements endowed with sense gradually emerged from it, they rendered it integrable. The work of decompression in analysis takes us down a similar path: the elements that emerge can be related to one another, to the analysand's experience, and hence integrated by him.

This work of differentiation is neither chronological nor gradual; it is more like the photographic process: the photographer uses different focal lengths to bring out coexistent planes that remain invisible while they are superimposed.

There is some danger in presenting the results of such differentiation in a book: on paper I may appear to bring out all the planes clearly and simultaneously, without showing that I was forced, with my patient, to change the adjustment and the focus time after time. In the course of analysis, one plane and one plane only seems clear at one time, though the analyst will remember that other planes continue to exist in blurred form.

Moreover, the clinical psychoanalyst will keep noting that the unconscious does not obey a temporal logic. During psychoanalysis, growing awareness does not follow a progressive chronology: highly evolved mechanisms can be discovered by the analysand before as well as after more regressive psychic mechanisms, or indeed at the same time. In any case, an act of awareness does not simply extend the list of previous acts of awareness; it modifies the entire psyche whose every component it changes; hence an analysand's discovery of how his vertigo relates to his oedipal conflicts may enable him to realize that he sometimes presents a form of vertigo involving the most regressive mechanisms.

The work of differentiation effected in the course of psychoanalysis is undoubtedly the counterpart of the work of condensation, used as a defence mechanism by the patient to ward off anxiety, or the instinctual forces and conflicts eliciting anxiety.

Naming the various forms of vertigo

During Luc's analysis, it emerged that each time a particular form of vertigo appeared, it assumed a special expression, corresponding to particular psychic mechanisms. In order to discover a meaning and representational value for each of these forms of vertigo, the better to get at its symbolic meaning, I felt that it was important for me to grasp its specific character, to the point of turning it into a distinct form of vertigo, to which I would give a specific name – just for myself. When I say that I named them *for myself*, that is because I never used these names with Luc or with any of my other patients. I used these names outside the sessions, in my work as a ruminating analyst, when I listened to the deep echoes of all the work done with such patients as Luc, so that I could feel the analytic process at work in the interaction of transference and counter-transference. It was not some arbitrary name that I assigned to each form of vertigo: to me, each name expressed the psychic mechanisms highlighted by this particular form of the symptom; it was my way of bringing to life the analytic space uniting Luc and myself. Luc, for his part, had no need to know the paths followed by my thought to feel our analytic space take on life and meaning.

All in all, I was thus led to name seven different vertigoes: fusion-related vertigo, vertigo related to being dropped, suction-related vertigo, imprison-ment/escape-related vertigo, vertigo related to attraction to the void, expansion-related vertigo, and competition-related vertigo. Characteristically, all these seven forms of vertigo appeared during Luc's analysis, and I also encountered them in my other patients. They correspond to my own under-standing of vertigo and serve me as useful reference points, but it is obvious that the presence of other forms of vertigo can be demonstrated equally well and that many other names could be coined.

At first, Luc believed that he suffered from just one form of vertigo: 'the' vertigo. It never even occurred to him that he might be suffering from sev-eral forms of vertigo because he always had the impression of having the same overall physical sensation: faintness coupled to a spinning sensation, though he could never tell whether he himself or his surroundings were spinning. He found this condition intolerable. Gradually, in the course of his analysis, or more precisely in Luc's experience of the interaction of trans-ference and counter-transference, his sensations became differentiated, hand in hand with the differentiation of the conditions under which these sensa-tions appeared and with his understanding of the corresponding psychic mechanisms. The clearer the differentiation, the more interested Luc became in representation and symbolization, and the less so in the vertigo sensation as such: learning to name the different forms of vertigo would have had no point for him; whereas I myself needed to name them to myself for the sake of Luc's analytic progress and for my own understanding of the process, because that was my way, as his analyst, of viewing them and of showing interest in them.

Notes

1 Psychoanalysts use the term *object* in a special sense, differing from that used in philosophy, grammar or in common speech. Segal defines it as follows: 'I think an object in the psychoanalytic sense is someone, or something, that has for us an emotional meaning. It is needed, or loved, hated or feared. Of necessity it is an object of perception' (1990: 49). However, other psychoanalysts use different definitions of the object, and Diatkine has stressed the danger of 'shifts in meaning that change this concept from object of a drive to that of object as opposed to subject' (1992: 67). In my view, the important thing about the object is to stress that to a very considerable extent the conception of it is built by the ego: 'The cathected object is not an image of the mother, or of the breast . . . but the direct result of the working over of a set of different experiences, inasmuch as it has developed in time, impinging jointly on the sensory functions, mobility, and the excitation of erogenous zones' (Diatkine 1992: 66).

2 By internal objects, I refer to phantasy representatives of persons important to the subject; the relationship between the ego and these internal objects would thus be the basis of the individual's psychic structure.

3 Freud never used the term 'decondensation' (*décondensation*). However, I have found it very helpful to make use of this term in French to designate the *reversal* of the process of condensation that Freud (1900a) described as one function of the dream-work. It is here translated as 'differentiation'.

2

Fusion-related vertigo

Anxiety about being destroyed together with the object

The most primitive form of the symptom

By *fusion-related vertigo* I refer to the most primitive type of the symptom, one that, so to speak, is the starting point of all the others. It is the vertigo of the patient who has the *sensation* that his legs are caving in, that he is sinking, that he is about to faint, and the *feeling* that he is about to disappear, to stop living. The patient is not afraid of falling, because the fear of falling presupposes that he continues to feel that he exists and that he is simply stumbling about in space or in the void. In fusion-related vertigo, he has on the one hand the feeling of being crushed and on the other hand no perception of space or of the void. He cannot fall into the void; he feels that he is disappearing on the spot.

Fortunately this extreme form of vertigo is rare – it is particularly painful. It corresponds to the distressed state of newly-born infants described by Freud as *Hilflosigkeit* (helplessness). Freud has shown that the distressed infant, if left to its own devices, is in danger on account of a *growing tension due to need,* against which it is helpless. ...the amounts of stimulation rise to an unpleasurable height without it being possible for them to be mastered psychically or discharged ...(Freud 1926d : 137). He went on to emphasize the imperative need of the infant for its mother or for a maternal substitute in the face of that threat.

> The emphasis placed on the danger of annihilation and the threat of overwhelming the ego is important because it means that the most regressive and psychotic reaction to separation probably arises because the fear of separation is equivalent to a fear of annihilation.
>
> (J.-M. Quinodoz 1993: 55)

The analysand suffering from fusion-related vertigo, and afraid of being

21

annihilated in a split-off part of himself, behaves rather like the distressed infant who has an absolute need of the object for his somatic and psychic survival. Clinical practice has shown that this type of analysand has a special need for the presence of the analyst, endowed with what Bion has called 'the mother's capacity for reverie' (Bion 1962: 36). The analyst's capacity for reverie plays an important role in helping the analysand to discover a meaning in his fusion-related vertigo.

This capacity for reverie is a form of primitive communication between mother and child, a communication consisting of projections and introjections which help the infant to discover his own feelings and thoughts. The infant projects into his mother what he cannot yet grasp about himself and what is therefore too frightening for him to integrate. The mother's capacity for reverie consists of her ability to accept what her infant has projected into her, to make sense of it, to find a solution, to transform it, in such a way that when she returns it to her child it will be de-dramatized enough and meaningful enough for the child to integrate and make use of it.

Most mothers use this capacity for reverie in a spontaneous and natural way. Let us imagine an infant is crying because he suddenly feels pangs he knows nothing about: his mother hears the child's cries, feels them in herself, and in her reverie imagines, for instance, that the child is feeling cold; she wraps him up in a blanket while telling him, even though he apparently still fails to make any sense of her words: 'You are cold, you'll feel better with this blanket.' The child then reintegrates an experience that makes sense twice over: it has both a direction (with a way out) and also a meaning. Next time he feels similar pangs, he can hope to make sense of it again. Moreover, since the content is inseparable from the ability to contain, the infant not only recovers what he has projected into his mother and what she has returned to him after having modified it herself, but also introjects the capacity of which his mother has given proof: her capacity for making sense of what she has received and for transforming it actively. In short, the infant introjects her capacity for thinking thoughts. In that way he comes to discover his own capacity to fulfil his needs, to think his thoughts and to direct his affects, in contact with the capacity of his mother which serves him, all in all, as an indispensable signpost.

Fusing with the object as a means of retaining it

When an analysand has been unable, in the regressive part of himself, to go beyond the primitive fear of being annihilated by separating himself from an important object, apparently essential to his survival, he may live in dread of such separation. He is suspicious of an object felt to be both essential and unreliable, and goes in constant fear that it may vanish. In that case he can use fusion as a mode of defence: in order to compel the object not to disappear, he can strive unconsciously to merge with it narcissistically in a part of his ego. It is rather as if he were saying to the object: 'I absorb you, I am you, there is no space between us, I can no longer lose you because we are "one"'.

This fusional object cannot be called a *containing* object, if we give that term a spatial or a symbolic meaning, because at that level there is no space – inside or out. In this regressive part of himself, the patient does not imagine that he could be contained in the object, but only that he might become fused with it.

Inasmuch as feeling a void arises from the feeling of having no object relations, we can say that this analysand *denies the void*; he is, in fact, denying the lack of communication with the object because he has the illusion of carrying the object with which he is fused wherever he goes. I am speaking of a denial, because in fusion the analysand does not take stock of psychic reality, namely the absence of an object relationship.

There can be a host of causes for this separation anxiety which, in turn, gives rise to the defence mechanism of fusion. The patient may have felt unable to rely on the presence of the object for what may seem to be good reasons: for example, he might have been deprived of this object at a very early age, or the object may not have been endowed with a sufficient capacity for reverie. However, in psychoanalysis, if we are to help the patient, we must above all consider his internal reality. Now, it should be noted that the construction of an internal object stable enough for the patient to tolerate separation from it depends not only on the capacity of the mother or her substitute, but also on the particular unconscious requirements of the child. A mother may, for instance, have an adequate capacity for reverie, but her child may be so envious of that maternal capacity that he destroys or misuses it unconsciously. That is why some patients who have had a disrupted childhood have nevertheless been able to construct stable internal objects, while others who have grown up securely in the midst of a stable family suffer grave separation anxiety.

Fusion may cause vertigo if the patient does not trust the object with which he is fused

The defence mechanism of fusion may not come into play should the analysand have the impression that the object with which he is fused is unreliable or likely to be destroyed. In that case, if he feels that the object is collapsing, he also gains the impression that he is collapsing with it, because in his phantasies the object and he are one. Now it is with an object felt to be unreliable that analysands presenting fusion-related vertigo have fused in a split-off part of their ego. I should like to make it clear that here I am not concerned with whether or not the object is reliable *in reality* (external reality); I am simply considering the internal object constructed by the analysand thanks to the constant interaction of his phantasies with his perceptions of the external world.

A case in point might be the vertigo of an analysand who has the impression that the lift carrying him is plunging down, is about to disintegrate and he *with* it; or the analysand whose legs give way *as if* the ground were caving in, so intimately fused is he, in his split-off part, with the lift or the ground; he feels that he is disappearing like the world fused with him. For these patients, in their split-off part, the lift or the ground are concrete equivalents of the unreliable object. Here I am referring to the *symbolic equation* introduced by Hanna Segal (1957). The lift and the ground do not *represent* the object, they do not *symbolize* it; they *are* the object in an equation replacing what might have been a symbol.

Luc's fusion-related vertigo – more frightening than I could ever have imagined

Luc was attacked by a striking form of fusion-related vertigo during his first analytic session and several times during the next few weeks. After that it never reappeared, except fleetingly when we agreed the date of the end of his analysis. Everything happened as if Luc had been able to integrate his most regressive anxieties quite rapidly thanks to the analyst's capacity for reverie. In the fusion-related vertigo that appeared during the first analytic session, Luc seemed glued to the couch, as if on the verge of physical and mental collapse and in the grip of immense anxiety, feeling absolutely rotten; his body tensed up, was convulsed with tremors, while some viscous substance was apparently being poured into his head. In short, he was experiencing the coenesthetic sensations that go with a mental block, something he had always feared might happen to him in his professional life.

In the course of the analysis, we were able to reconstruct that occasion, that is the time when Luc lay down on my couch that first time and hence lost sight of me. I had become a childhood object, evanescent and judged to be unreliable but nevertheless essential to his sense of being alive, so much so that it became essential for him to hang on to me. Unconsciously, he had incorporated me, fused with me, so that we could not be separated: for Luc, my presence was reduced to his sensation of being glued to the couch.

However, as in his phantasies, once out of sight, I became an unreliable transference object, liable to being destroyed. I was disappearing from him in two senses: I was out of his view and I was also annihilated. Because he was fused with me in his regressive part, he disappeared and collapsed with me. In that regressive moment, Luc made a symbolic equation between the analyst and the couch. For him, in his split-off part, I was the couch that collapsed, and he, Luc, collapsed *with* the couch, being fused with it as he was with myself.

Defence by projective identification

Vertigo projected into the analyst

In the transference, infraverbal communication of a primitive kind by projective identification was so pronounced that, in the session preceding the first weekend of Luc's analysis, I experienced vertigo myself. That weekend was our first separation and evoked unspeakable primitive anxieties in Luc. For my part, I felt the room sway about me and clung tightly to my armchair, a response that took me aback for a moment before I realized, in my counter-transference, that this was a projection of Luc into myself. As soon as I grasped that my vertigo had come not from me but from Luc, and that I could use it to understand what Luc was feeling and hence to communicate with him, the vertigo stopped.

In our transference/counter-transference, Luc and I were engaged in a communication of the same type as that described by Bion in connection with the mother's capacity for reverie. Luc himself was unable to integrate the vertiginous anxiety he felt and hence he unconsciously projected it into me so that I might make sense of it and help him to integrate it. In relying on my own feelings, I was able to put into words his feeling that his ego and the object were collapsing, as reflected in his feelings that the room was collapsing – all of it connected with my disappearance during this first weekend.

Naming the different types of vertigo to nail down the terror

I fully realized, during that session, what great dangers lie in wait for the analyst in this primitive communication. I might have felt anxious about Luc's anxiety which had such effects on me, and have refused to put up with his projections; but in that case my anxiety would have been added to Luc's which he would then have had to reproject into me with redoubled force, thus increasing my own anxiety: we should have been drawn into a more and more inextricable spiral of a *folie à deux*. 'If the mother cannot tolerate these projections, the infant is reduced to continued projective identification with increasing force and frequency. The increased force seems to denude the projection of its penumbra of meaning' (Bion 1967: 115). Luc would then have built me up as an internal object thus robbing me of my capacity to understand him, which would have contributed to undermining his own potential to grasp his anxieties.

I might equally well have worried about nothing but my own vertigo and have failed to consider that it might stem from Luc's anxiety projected into myself. That would have been tantamount to rejecting his projection and leaving him to cope with his distress by himself. In that case, Luc's anxiety would have rebounded on him without my having given it any meaning; Luc would then have felt that his vertigo was quite senseless. Luc's vertigo would have reflected his fear of annihilation; he would have found himself in the situation described by Bion: that of a mother unable to accept the projection into herself of the infant's feeling that it is dying, so much so that 'the infant feels that its feeling that it is dying is stripped of such meaning as it has. It therefore reintrojects, not a fear of dying made tolerable but a nameless dread' (Bion 1967: 116). Bion's 'nameless dread' struck me as being a highly suggestive term. The most intolerable anxiety is that which has no name because it has no meaning; the moment we begin to give it a meaning, we can name the dread or the anxiety. I then realized how important it was for me to assign names to Luc's various types of vertigo as they began to make sense in the analysis: they then became different *forms of dread with a name*.

However, I was not immune to another mistake: I might be wrong about the meaning of the projections I had received from my patient and, drawing on my own experience, have offered interpretations more or less remote from his. But that is a risk run by all mothers who use their capacity for reverie. Such mistakes are not only inevitable but indispensable, because they prove that there is a difference between mother and child. They are the faults in the communication that elicit a reaction from the child and encourage it to start correcting the mother's responses. The essential thing is that the analyst, or the mother, should accept a margin of uncertainty as something positive.

I have always been moved by the character of the nurse in Jean Anouilh's tragedy, *Antigone*. At the beginning of the play, the nurse, who took charge of Antigone and Ismene on the death of their mother Jocasta, is deeply distressed because she has failed to prevent Antigone and her sister from leaving the house in the night and because she cannot understand what might have drawn them outside. The nurse never imagined that Antigone or her sister might have suffered fears whose origin was not connected with their basic needs; that is why in dealing with the problems of her 'little ones' she was always ready to come up with the same simple solutions, for instance, slices of buttered bread, hot milk or a woolly sweater; at a pinch she could imagine that a love affair was involved. And the nurse goes on to imagine Jocasta's reproaches to her:

'Spend your life making them behave, watching over them like a mother hen, running after them with mufflers and sweaters to keep them warm and eggnogs to make them strong and then at four o'clock in the morning, you who always complained you could never sleep a wink, snoring in your bed and letting them slip out in the bushes . . .'

(1951: 16)

I feel that the nurse's distress reflects her sudden realization that she had allowed routine to put the inventiveness of her capacity for reverie to sleep. It may sometimes seem very reassuring for a nursing mother to tell herself, from force of habit, that her infant is crying because he is hungry! But here we have a nurse realizing that Antigone's last displays of agony had a complex significance which had escaped her, and that the usual solutions were far from adequate. As an analyst I feel close to that nurse, because I know how important it is to keep one's capacity for reverie alive, and to be careful not to reuse interpretations even if they have proved adequate in the past. All the same, the analyst, like the nurse, may not to be wide awake at four o'clock in the morning... No doubt the psychoanalyst must therefore accept the possibility of failure despite his or her habitual vigilance, so that the analysand may feel that, when all is said and done, it is up to him to watch over his own life.

Excessive projective identification

Luc's projection of his vertigo into the analyst with whom he identified himself narcissistically can be considered an example of *projective identification* (Klein 1946); in this case, it was the kind of projective identification said to be *excessive*, inasmuch as Luc made unconscious use of this defence mechanism mainly as discharge and not as a means of communication.

When there is strong aggression in a split-off part of the patient's ego it may be very important that the analyst, paying very careful heed to the counter-transference, should make positive use of this excessive projective identification, verbalize it and turn it into a means of communication. This may sometimes prevent the patient from making unconscious use of excessive projective identification, not merely with the analyst but also with his own family. Now, there may be a particular danger if he uses it with his family because, generally, they are unable to decode his projections and hence to treat them as attempts at communication. Family members pose the threat of colluding with the patient, that is, of failing to realize that these projections come from the patient and believing instead that they come from themselves. It has been known, for instance, that a patient who had great difficulty in containing his impulse to fling himself into the void had the distressing experience of seeing a member of his family, with whom he had a very close narcissistic relationship, jump out of a window when nothing suggested he was likely to do so. Luckily, he was not seriously hurt; bit by bit the analysand was able to discover what had happened: he had unconsciously and forcefully projected his anxiety and his impulse to jump into space into the other person; the latter had mistaken this projection for his own anxiety and impulse and had then acted in the patient's stead.

Fusion-related vertigo and separation anxiety

Two of Luc's episodes of acting-out later made it possible to gain a clearer picture of the link between the disappearance of the object and the appearance of fusion-related vertigo. On two occasions, meeting me elsewhere than in the waiting room where he usually saw me, Luc collapsed on the spot. Referring to this response during the sessions, he told me that when he saw me where he had not expected me to be, his image of myself had collapsed and he with it. *There was no longer even an empty space* into which he could drop. If I disappeared, he disappeared. We were close to the concept of the flat two-dimensional space discussed by Bick (1968) and Meltzer (1975) in connection with adhesive identification.

Moreover, at the time, Luc never spoke to me about what happened between analytic sessions. It was his highly regressive split-off part that he chiefly brought to analysis, and here nothing seemed to exist for him other than the fused state in which he had the illusion that we were joined together beyond space and time. When I speak of a fused state, I am referring to an asymptotic condition; in fact, I consider fusion as the phantasy of an unattainable illusory state, towards which we can tend by an asymptotic process whose extreme representation would be fusion in the void. Indeed, if fusion were ever attained, the fused objects would be destroyed because they would forfeit their differences and hence their existence as distinct and irreplaceable persons.

We can now see what threats fusion can pose to the analysand. It can seem fascinating, as it did to Luc, but at the same time it can also seem dreadful. When a patient has nothing but this fused mode as his image of possible relationships, he may suffer from permanent anxiety: in fact, outside the fusion there is only the void because there are no relationships, and in the fusion there is annihilation because the person disappears. For a patient to emerge from fusion, it is not enough that he defuse himself from the object with which he has been fused; he must also discover a mode of relationship other than the fused, that is, a mode of object relationship. Luc will give us occasion to return to this topic.

The wish for fusion reflected in speech

Luc translated his desire to be *at one* with me by the way he spoke to me during the sessions. In fact, at the beginning of the analysis, during moments close to fusion-related vertigo, Luc reeled off words in a monotonous voice, slowly and in a whisper, while delivering interminable monologues without any obvious logical connection, apparently addressing me not as a distinct interlocutor, but as an interlocutor situated within himself. He made me feel that he was addressing me through himself, as if the two of us were amalgamated. Why should he have raised his voice or verbalized his complete chain of thoughts when, in his phantasy, I was fused with him, when my thoughts were fused with his, and hence so familiar to me that he had no need to put them into words for me? Sometimes a sentence begun would be completed in silence, as if Luc was certain that I would continue to hear it to the end.

I had the impression that what Luc was repeating during the analysis, by his way of speaking to me, was his wish to be part of me, so that I might never separate myself from him. I considered this quest for fusion a sign of unconscious aggression towards me, inasmuch as, without realizing it, he was trying by it to force me to stick with him, not to think differently from him, to deprive me of my freedom to be different from him, in short preventing me from being myself. When I tried to interpret the meaning of his manner of speaking, the mere sound of my voice, breaking the illusion of our fusion, unleashed fusion-related vertigo in Luc. The very fact that my voice came from the outside was a shocking demonstration to Luc that I was not inside him and thus, escaping from his control, threatening to disappear. Nevertheless, if Luc used this way of speaking with me, in the same way as his other manifestations of anxiety, it was surely so that, in the analysis, we could assign some meaning to it and work it over.

References to castration that actually lead back to a more regressive anxiety

Despite its apparent incoherence, Luc's discourse during that phase of the analysis enabled me to get slightly closer to the contents of the phantasies connected with the physical sensations he expressed. Luc, his eyes shut, saw very garish and unconnected images which he listed: necks of disembodied chickens, cut-up rabbits, broken motor-car spanners . . . These images, which had no meaning for Luc, suggested castration anxiety to me. As Luc listed these images in a dramatic way, his tensed-up body was shaken by uncontrollable tremors. In order to put an end to these frightening scenes, I was forced not only to verbalize the symbolic castration significance of the material he brought me, but also to offer myself as a castrated object. For

29

example: 'When you see all those cut-up objects isn't it perhaps as if you saw me with a cut-off penis and were afraid that might actually have happened to me.'

Several conditions were therefore needed to render Luc's anxiety more able to be integrated:

- naming the danger by closing off the detour of the symbolic equation: chicken necks made way for cut-off penises;
- presenting myself as the castrated object, which helped Luc to get out of the narcissistic confusion: it was me and not himself he had seen castrated in his phantasies; we were therefore different and, in the space created between us, there was room for feelings; with my formulation ('You were afraid . . .') I had discreetly suggested the possibility that he might be solicitous about me while feeling disturbed about a threat to himself;
- to verbalize these two aspects together, thus showing that, to me, it was all a phantasy which we could examine together and not a dramatic objective reality.

My use of the words 'castration' and 'penis' may wrongly suggest that I focused my interpretations on a genital level of the libido. In fact, the phantasy expressed by Luc during his enumeration of cut-up objects while his whole body was shaking was highly regressive: Luc took his entire body for a part object: a penis. His fusion-related vertigo went hand in hand with moments of physical frenzy – during the sessions, a part of Luc's ego behaved as if his entire body was a penis in danger of being castrated and destroyed by fusion with an object that seemed to him on the point of collapse.

I hesitated for a long time before first interpreting Luc's recourse to the part object. I imagined he would take me for a perfect idiot, get up and walk out. What was sometimes difficult for me to bear in mind was to what point the part of Luc that addressed itself to me had regressed, and that I had to be very careful when expressing it in the appropriate terms. I found myself again clinging to my armchair (just as I had done when I myself had succumbed to the vertigo induced by Luc) when I told him: 'When you shake all over your body while telling me about those cut-off objects, you may perhaps be feeling like a great big penis trembling with anxiety at the thought that it is in danger of being cut off.' Luc was not shocked; this kind of language obviously got through to him. After a long silence he said calmly: 'Now I understand why I have the impression that a viscous fluid fills my head; I was putting sperm into it!' From then on, Luc could give free rein to his corporeal phantasies, because he guessed that his physical sensations might correspond to representations and to phantasies.

I think that before we can refer usefully to a genital libido, the penis must represent a component of the total object in the corporeal phantasy image; for as long as the penis is phantasized as a part object – whether or not it is taken for the whole – the anxiety proves to be more regressive and the libido to be pregenital. I believe that we must distinguish a *total* object from a *global* object; they occur on two different levels. The total object is structured, personalized and opposed to the part object; the global object is not structured and may be a part object mistaken for a whole. I shall be returning to this point; in Luc's phantasy, the body was a global part object.

Splitting

I believe that the reason why Luc stopped complaining of fusion-related vertigo, following my interpretation of his tremors, was largely that, by verbalizing what happened in his *mad* part, I had rendered it intelligible to his *adjusted* part, thus giving Luc reason to hope that he might be able to reduce the split between these two parts of himself. Through the impression, in my counter-transference, that Luc was going to treat me as a fool and leave me, I had felt Luc's internal conflict inside myself. I was the spokesman of that incomprehensible part of Luc which his adjusted part considered to be mad and of which he hoped to rid himself. My interpretation, conferring a meaning upon the manifestations of that split-off part, helped to strip it of its magically omnipotent character: its meaning began to dawn on him and the split-off part no longer seemed so alien to Luc. He could start to treat it as part of himself, even though he could not yet integrate it.

However, before that could happen, Luc had not only to introject the content of the interpretation, he had also to introject the analyst's capacity to take care of his *mad* part and to adopt it. He discovered that he himself could continue the interpretation and discover a meaning in the phantasies of that part of himself which might become an aspect of his ego.

At the preliminary interviews, when Luc had spoken about his impressions of collapsing as if they had happened to a stranger, I had resisted taking cognizance of the split, because unconsciously I had paid attention to Luc's manifest expectations and not to his latent and profound demand: for him it went without saying that I was bound to be the ally of that part of himself which was adjusted to reality.

The beginnings of thought

Fusion-related vertigo relates to the first sensations that enabled each one of us to construct an inner space inseparable from the corporeal ego and constituting the early beginnings of thought. In this connection, my attention was drawn to what Haag had to say about the foundations of thought:

> We are led to consider the nature of the first emotional exchanges underlying the transformation of sensations into perceptions and thought. But are not the first emotions themselves supported by sensations that become organized during the instinctual encounter? That is how the first ideograms are formed.
>
> (Haag 1991a: 51)

I might equally well have referred to Anzieu, according to whom the first thought initially organizes the corporeal ego and space: the formal signifiers as Anzieu defines them 'fall into the general category of representatives of things, more particularly of representatives of space and of bodies in general' (Anzieu 1987).

Haag was forced to invent terms for conveying these early, non-verbalized experiences involved in the construction of an internal space inherent in the corporeal ego experienced as having a base and a direction, and from which thought emerges. She insists, for instance, on the role of the 'attentive look' and above all on the importance of the 'concomitance of the tactile experience of dorsal contact and the interpretation of looks' (Haag, 1991b). This concomitance allows the construction of the first 'sensation-sentiments' of 'background-space with a bottom' which helps to 'surmount the panic fears of the exploration of the depth of outer space'.

The situation Haag describes is something I have encountered myself especially in analysands with fusion-related vertigo. Much of what I have observed in these patients began to make sense in the light of her remarks; in particular, I must stress the importance of the 'attentive look' I exchanged with them the moment we found ourselves in the waiting room. It seemed evident to me that this exchange of looks, in which our presence and our mutual attention were concentrated, is continued by the patients during the session, and that they associate it with the intense 'sensation-sentiment' of the supine position, the back quite flat, corresponding to the search for a space with a bottom. These patients generally keep their eyes shut as they concentrate on what is happening within them. I believe that the combination or coincidence of this inward look and feeling their back enables them to rediscover the 'sensation-sentiment' of the small infant who has his back firmly supported by the person carrying him, which constitutes a basis for the emergence of thought.

3

Vertigo related to being dropped

Anxiety about being dropped by the object

When Luc's analysis had reached a more advanced stage, my interventions into his fusion-related speech no longer elicited fusion-related vertigo, but another form of vertigo, which I have called *vertigo related to being dropped*. This second type of vertigo had made itself felt in earlier sessions as well but had been masked by the more invasive fusion-related type.

In his vertigo related to being dropped, Luc no longer had the impression that he was collapsing *with* the couch but that he was falling *from* the couch *into* the void; he was not being destroyed with the couch, but felt that he had been dropped from it. Uncontrolled movements and coenesthetic sensations had ceased. Luc defended himself from the danger of losing the divan-object no longer by *fusing* with it, but by *clinging* to it. This act reminded me of my own clinging to the armchair when I had felt invaded by Luc's projections of vertiginous anxiety: at the time I had unconsciously modified those projections as soon as I received them, transforming into a clinging mechanism what had still been fusional in Luc's case. I had thus come to realize to what a large extent the receiving object impresses his personal stamp on the projections he receives in projective identification.

Luc was intimately familiar with vertigo related to being dropped in everyday life: it was the vertigo he experienced when he had the impression that lifts or cable-cars were about to open up and let him fall out.

Vertigo related to being dropped: separation and differentiation

I was able to observe that the onset of this type of vertigo during analysis appeared in some patients at certain strategic moments of separation, for instance on the announcement that the session was over or just before the vacations. In this connection I would recall that, as early as 1914, Ferenczi mentioned the vertigo or giddiness experienced at the end of the psycho-analytic session. He said that the explanation that this vertigo was the result of the sudden change from the recumbent position to the sitting position struck him as a rationalization. In his view, this type of vertigo was 'an example of the manner in which psychic states of excitement overflow into the bodily sphere'; he also thought that, in fact, the patient finds it extremely difficult to keep his balance as he moves from one psychic situation to the next: at the end of the sessions the patient feels 'as though fallen from the clouds', is stripped of his illusions as he realizes that

> it is the paid doctor and not the helpful father that stands before him . . . The patient who a moment before unreservedly revealed his most inti-mate secrets now confronts the doctor as a 'stranger' before whom he thinks he should be and actually is ashamed, like someone discovering that his clothes are not properly 'buttoned up'.
>
> (1914: 240–241)

In short the patient feels deserted by the psychoanalyst.

In any case, with patients subject to vertigo related to being dropped, the symptom is triggered off by moments of differentiation: one of these may be the end of the session but there are a good many others as well. For exam-ple, there was a period when Luc experienced vertigo related to being dropped every time I interrupted one of his fusion-related monologues: when Luc addressed me as someone fused with him, my interruption demonstrated that I existed outside him and was therefore distinct from him; it was then that vertigo related to being dropped appeared. This shows in particular that there is a link between this type of vertigo and the threat of losing the object by differentiation from it.

The object seemingly dropping the patient

The feelings accompanying vertigo related to being dropped are highly characteristic. During spells of this type of vertigo, an analysand might well think of me as an analyst with no personal interest in the patient, someone only concerned with him out of a sense of duty or because he takes great care not to say or do anything the analyst might seize upon as a pretext for 'dropping him'.

The end of every session can thus seem like a moment when the analyst drops the patient into the void: once the door is shut behind him, the patient imagines that he no longer exists for the analyst, the discontinuity of the relationship entailing the discontinuity of the object. These transference feelings often go back to the phantasy that the parents want nothing so much as to get rid of their children and that they forget all about them as soon as they see that the children, absorbed in some interesting occupation, take their eyes off them. Analysands can reproduce this oedipal phantasy during analysis, for example not daring to do anything interesting during the analyst's vacation, or not daring to tell the analyst that they did do this or that for fear that the analyst might take advantage of it to increase the distance between them ('Seeing that the analysand takes my absence so well, I'll profit from it in the future!'); or to decide that the patient no longer needs analysis ('Since the patient does not complain, I shall take advantage of the situation and turn my attention elsewhere!'). This is reminiscent of Spitz's descriptions of 'abandonic' children.

The act of clinging to the couch corresponds to the unconscious attempt to cling to the analyst; the analysand can, for instance, make a point of never missing a single second of a session, as if he had to make absolutely certain that the analyst was there and not ready to drop him; he may phantasize that the analyst cannot possibly be elsewhere than in his armchair between sessions, to which end he must immobilize the analyst in his thoughts lest the analyst escape; he must never take the risk of annoying the analyst, of contradicting him, or of showing that he is different from him, thus not giving him the least excuse for abandoning the patient.

These psychic mechanisms sometimes stand in the way of the patient's creativity, and hence of the success of his analysis. They can bring home to us all the unconscious aggression implicit in the look of the analysand who cannot help seeing his analyst as an indifferent, insensitive being, one for whom the analysand does not count. The analysand rarely realizes that this look can affect his analyst; however it usually does, even though the analyst is perfectly aware that, in the transference, this look is not addressed to him directly. Actually, it is very important that the analyst should be affected, because counter-transference affects are indispensable for grasping what the analysand is trying to express.

The wish to drop the analysand in the counter-transference

The material Luc brought to me threw light on my counter-transference, and showed me that whenever Luc was seized by vertigo related to being dropped during the analysis, he was using projective identification with greater than usual force to communicate with me: in fact, despite Luc's assiduous attendance of his analytic sessions and his declared wish to continue with them, I had been feeling doubts for some time about my ability to carry his analysis *to its term* and had had scruples about continuing with it. These scruples even made me feel that, because of my doubts in my own

35

competence, it would be more honest to tell Luc that I preferred to break off the analysis.

Luckily, realizing that Luc himself had not the least wish to cut the analysis short, I tried to get to the bottom of my feeling that I was incapable of going on with this analysis. Had it originated with me? Did it really reflect my own inadequacy? That conclusion seemed bizarre to me, the more so as, with my other ongoing analyses I readily accepted that I was not omnipotent and that I could do no more than try my best; I simply expected my patients to make good use of what help I could offer them so that they could get on with their own analysis. Why then did I discover a different attitude in my dealings with this particular analysand? Did this attitude originate with Luc? Did Luc once again display a defence mechanism through projective identification with its double character of *identification* and *projection*? Did this phantasy and the feelings it elicited spring from Luc; did he *project* them into me by *narcissistic identification*, which allowed him to link his identity to this phantasy and to these feelings, because they were *projected* into another self of his?

I then realized that Luc was so intensely afraid of having an internal mother set on having an abortion that I ended up feeling in my countertransference the affects corresponding to the role into which he had cast me in his phantasy, namely that of a mother who feels unable to carry her pregnancy to its full term. Had I really cut Luc's analysis short, I should have *acted out* and realized Luc's phantasy instead of interpreting it, that is, I should have given him proof that I was in fact, just as in his phantasy, an analyst-mother who interrupts the ongoing creative process. However, having discovered the meaning of what Luc was projecting into me, I was able to reconstruct the phantasy with Luc instead of acting it out. I did not, of course, tell Luc what I had felt, nor make him privy to the course of my thoughts, but helped him to rediscover his phantasy, which had been at the root of what I had felt. The reconstruction of that phantasy brought back a screen memory: Luc remembered that his mother had told him in very harsh detail that while she was pregnant with him she had tried to have an abortion. In analysis, he rediscovered the anxiety of being dropped by the maternal womb (part object) or by the mother (whole object); he realized that he was repeating this feeling in the analysis through the fear that I might 'drop him from the analysis' if he did not hold on tight. This enabled us later to interpret in the transference the conflict and the aggressive phantasies involving a son and a mother destroying each other.

Don Juan and the Princess in A Thousand and One Nights

The patient who feels that the important object is constantly about to drop him sometimes unconsciously adopts an attitude of mirroring in his analysis: he treats the analyst as if he, the patient, were about to drop him. It is with analysands using a Don Juan approach that I have most often experienced the transference and counter-transference swings in which the analysand gives the analyst the feeling that he is about to let go of him, that feeling being the stronger the more the analysand originally produced extremely rich analytic material designed to seduce the analyst. In fact, these patients who present themselves to their analysts with an impressive catalogue of all the women they have seduced and abandoned repeat in their dealings with the analyst, treated as their mother, a constant script of seduction and abandonment. That scenario is often an unconscious projection of what the patient felt with his mother during early infancy: 'Everything happens as if the patient wanted to re-enact with a woman the role he was once forced to play himself: that of being seduced and abandoned' (D. Quinodoz 1986: 1005).

I do not wish to enter into the various processes that lead the Don Juan-analysand to repeat the process of seduction and abandonment in the transference with the analyst-mother, or to repeat with the analyst-father his feeling of exasperation with the intruder (as if the patient were trying unconsciously to be thrown out by the analyst-father); all I do want to stress here is that the resulting counter-transference response can be summed up by my impression that the analyst-mother finds herself in the situation of the Princess in *A Thousand and One Nights* who says:

> I have a date with a man who wants unconsciously to take revenge, through me, on the woman who, he felt, abandoned him after she seduced him. Every session is a night in which I must keep my head if I want the analysis to continue; to do that, a story has to be told at every session, but not just any story: the only story capable of fascinating Don Juan enough for him to renounce his desire to do away with me is his own story, that of his suffering, of his feeling abandoned, of his narcissistic wound. What I have to do is to put it into words by means of what we re-experience together in the thousand and one facets of the transference, so that he may at last be able to imagine, to picture for himself and to verbalize that early wound which has proved so ineffable.
>
> (D. Quinodoz 1986: 1007–8)

Comparison with fusion-related vertigo: the emergence of the sense of the void

If we compare this form of vertigo with fusion-related vertigo, we shall find that, in vertigo related to being dropped, the object is not felt to *collapse* but to be *letting go* of one. There is no fusion of the ego with the object, and we can begin to speak of a containing object. Even though what we have here is still a very simple concept of a container (the original phantasy involving a passive content), it already presupposes a differentiation between container and contained and between inside and out. Moreover, the distinction between object and ego must persist even during vertigo if the containing object is to be felt as dropping what it contains.

This means that, in analysis, the analyst is felt to be liable to *drop* his analysand *into the void*. It is no longer a case of two fused objects disappearing together. The notion of the void expressing the absence of the object relation is no longer denied as it is in vertigo related to fusion. The separation anxiety becomes more conscious and more harrowing, because the analysand no longer has the illusion of dragging along an analyst to whom he is fused wherever he goes. The very presence of the analyst can then be felt to be harrowing because he is thought of as a 'dropping' analyst. This type of patient seems to be reacting more sharply to the separation than a patient fused with his analyst, but that does not mean that his separation anxiety is more intense – far from it. J.-M. Quinodoz has shown that 'the apparent absence of a reaction conceals excessive anxiety' (1993: 10), and that, as a result, separation anxiety is particularly acute in patients who are not conscious of their reactions to the separation. They present great distress in various ways but cannot say why, while patients who are conscious of suffering from a separation see a reason for their anguish and are able to make better use of it in shaping their lives.

Much the same happens with vertigo: vertigo related to fusion gives rise to annihilation anxiety, the analysand having a sense of existential destruction; moreover the object is not felt to have been lost but to be non-existent. In vertigo related to being dropped subject and object both continue to exist, the subject suffering because he has the feeling that the object is about to drop him and that he, the patient, is about to lose the object.

From the feeling of void to the feeling of space and from symbolic equation to symbol

Abandoning fusion for the void or for relational space?

Daring to take the risk

How can the patient come to realize that if he takes the risk of abandoning the fusional relationship with his analyst (which can elicit fusion-related vertigo) he will not be left with a relational void (which can trigger off vertigo related to being dropped) but will still be able to establish object relations whose quality warrants the trouble of taking a risk? How does the analysand proceed from the feeling of anxiety – 'The analyst has separated himself from me to drop me into the void' – to a feeling of hope: 'The analyst has let go of me so that the two of us might create object relations in relational space'? Now it is the transition from the first to the second feeling which allows the analysand to go on with his analysis.

Analysis encourages the construction of relational space

I believe that analysis has a specific characteristic that encourages the transformation of the space of separation into object-linking space: this characteristic springs from the *concomitance* of (1) the analytic setting and (2) the work of psychoanalytic interpretation.

The analytic setting is indispensable because it reflects the recognition that the analyst is a person distinct from the analysand, that he has his own limits and his own needs, without which he would cease to function as an analyst.

> By proposing a precise setting, namely the analytic setting, to his patient, the analyst states the conditions he needs in order to function as an analyst, and especially the conditions specifying the time, the psychic rather than acting-out character of the sessions, and also the payment of the fees. These are so many limitations defining the analyst's work and against which the analysand may come up the better to discover his own ways. It may happen that the narcissistic analysand, having fusional tendencies, will attack the setting, that he will try desperately to convince the analyst to act differently, to renounce his own ways and to conform with the analysand's. It may also happen that he welcomes the setting and adheres to it in a fusional way. In both cases he has a tendency to obliterate the psychic space of separation which permits the use of symbolization, acting as if that space were bound to be a gulf.
>
> (D. Quinodoz 1989c: 1650)

This narcissistic attitude is quite different from that of a patient who, respecting the form of the proposed analytic setting, finds that it does not suit him and that he would rather look for another style of treatment.

If the setting was all there was, it might indeed be taken for a barrier, because it would only be a negative aspect of the process of differentiation and not part of the search for communication. The statement 'I am eager to distinguish myself from you' would be presented without its justification: 'because that is essential if we are to communicate'. Moreover, at the beginning of the analysis, the patient will sometimes feel that the demands of the setting are castrating or rejecting constraints; in that case the analyst will strike him as a severe internal object (super-ego) in the transference, and the

39

patient will be only too ready to hear the inevitable announcement of the end of the session as: 'I am dropping you because the hour is up, we have agreed on this contractually, and you have ceased to exist for me until the next session.'

Combining setting and interpretation

In analysis, the setting ensuring the separation of analyst and analysand is combined with the work of interpretation by which analyst and patient can confront their limits. Without the constraints of the setting, the interpretation might appear to be dangerous and invasive; conversely, without the interpretation and the consequent confrontation of the respective limits, the setting might open up a gulf between the analysand and the analyst. The whole process reflects the analyst's particular way of listening to the patient during the analysis, which allows the confrontation of the analyst's approach with the analysand's. In fact, in this form of listening, the analysand discovers that his comments are thrown back at him by the analyst in a way that is both similar to and different from his own, inasmuch as by 'reflecting' his comments, the analyst reveals their latent, unconscious, meaning, that is, what the analysand has put into them without realizing that he has done so.

This process helps the analysand to realize that there is a space in which the analyst's and his own propositions, while different, may often be connected by a link springing from the unconscious, and previously hidden from the patient. This process of interpretation which enables the analysand to see a connection, where he originally saw nothing but the void, helps him to realize that strict acceptance of the setting, on which the analyst keeps insisting, may not be the analyst's way of rejecting him, but of maintaining the conditions indispensable for the possible appearance of an object-relational space. 'For the analysand this constitutes the experience that the pleasure of establishing connections may prevail over the fear of a possible rupture' (D. Quinodoz 1989c: 1651).

The analyst upsets the analysand's fusional illusion

In any case, the double thrust 'I separate myself from you so that we might be connected (if each one of us should desire it)' is of great importance to patients suffering from fusion-related vertigo or from vertigo related to being dropped. Now, the analyst seems inordinately cruel to his patients every time he dwells on their separation, and he may well be tempted, for the sake of peace and greater convenience, to leave the patient with the illusion that fusion can be achieved.

40

The analyst might, for instance, make it a point never to interrupt the patient's interminable fusional monologues and retire behind a wall of silence or the so-called neutrality of the analyst. The analysand seemingly wants nothing better. The analyst may also not stand firm and fail to insist on certain conditions of the setting that the analysand rejects in the course of the analysis, because they over-emphasize the differences between his own wishes and the analyst's. This might reduce tensions, but would mean colluding with the analysand and leaving him under the illusion that the analyst is willing to meet his fusional desires. Now, the analysand, despite his manifest wishes, needs the analyst to ignore them, and would be able to bear it all the better if the analyst brought home to him the two terms of the differentiation: to demonstrate the distance between them the better to bridge it.

From symbolic equation to the non-equation that makes symbolism possible

In order to verbalize the phantasies accompanying vertigo related to being dropped which Luc experienced while lying on the couch, he invoked sensations linked to bodily images. One day, after one of my interventions bringing out the differences between us, Luc had the impression that the couch on which he was lying had let go of him, and exclaimed: 'I can feel the cable-car opening under me like a womb dropping me'. That phrase struck me as being important because it made me realize that Luc, in this regressive part of himself, was still using the symbolic *equation*, even while beginning to allow for a *non-equation* capable of further opening the door to symbolism. In fact, the moment Luc gained the feeling during the session that I had dropped him, the analyst *was* (equation) the couch, which *was* the cable-car, but which was *like* (non-equation) a womb.

When two objects are equated, they are equivalent, interchangeable; there is no space between them allowing differentiation and a developed symbolism. There is merely a rudimentary form of a still very concrete symbolism. In the scheme of symbolic equations, objects are either equated, that is confused, or else they are not, that is, they are simply juxtaposed without being correlated; between them there is no relational space, but only the absence of relations, a void which, moreover, is sometimes denied. By contrast, once there is similarity or non-equation marked by the use of the word *like*, the objects are seen to be distinct rather than identical; though their similarities are brought out, they nevertheless remain different and a relational space between them is possible.

For Hanna Segal, the symbolic equation, which is a primitive form of symbolization, is the basis of the concrete thought characteristic of psychosis (1957); she stresses that it is in the depressive position, when there is a greater degree of differentiation and separation between the ego and the object, that symbols can be used to compensate for object losses. The concept of symbolic equation is extremely valuable; however, one must take care with the use of the adjective *symbolic* in this expression; in fact, this qualifier can cause confusion since it is precisely the *equation* of objects which prevents the introduction of an advanced symbolic activity; the equation is, so to speak, used instead of what might have been a symbol in the strict sense of the term and is merely a sketch of a symbol.

Part objects juxtaposed in the void or whole objects correlated in space

One of the aims of my interventions with analysands suffering from vertigo related to being dropped is to help them create a relational space between them and the object that is increasingly open to symbolism. This facilitates a gradual advance from part objects *juxtaposed* in the *void* to total objects *correlated* in space. I should like to recall that these patients suffering from vertigo related to being dropped do not present regressive defence mechanisms except in a part, or in a more or less important facet, of their ego, and that the rest of their personality remains quite open to symbolism. To return to Luc's case, he had me go on from *one* formulation of the order of the symbolic equation in which 'I was' my consulting room, which 'was' the cable-car, which 'was' my womb; to formulations in which, for Luc, 'being in my room was *like* being in the cable-car *threatening* to open up beneath him', or, again, '*as if* my room might be my womb, and as if he, Luc, *might be* the child I carried *inside me* and *might* drop'. In these new formulations I no longer *was* my room, the couch or the cable-car, but was being *represented* by them (resembled them) with the possibility of being symbolized by them.

We can see that the abandonment of the symbolic equation goes hand in hand with the introduction not only of the distinction between the terms of the equation (analyst, couch, cable-car) but also between the patient and the object with whom he maintained a fusional relationship. In fact, the analyst is no longer the couch, which is no longer the cable-car, so that he finds it harder to fuse with the analyst – he is no longer prepared to fuse with the couch or with the cable-car in order to be with the analyst. At the same time, however, another important point arises: the concept of *non-equation* entailing the notion of space between objects, so that we can go on to speak of their respective positions as well as of inside and outside (for example, in his phantasies, Luc could feel like a child *in* my womb). Now that feeling which, in its turn, entails the idea of proceeding from the inside to the outside, or vice versa, introduces an element of uncertainty or risk and hence of freedom ('I can drop the child in my womb voluntarily or otherwise but

I can also keep it'). As soon as the possibility of freedom is introduced, the entire quality of the relationship is changed. In Luc's new formulation, it was 'as if I was *a mother* (and no longer a womb) and as if he was the child I was *expecting* (and no longer the one I carry)'. I was no longer the part object, either in the fragmented form in which I was nothing but a womb, or in the global form of mother-womb in which the part is taken for the whole. The alternative formulation designates the analyst as a whole person, a psychic presence, a synthesis of different aspects of himself or herself, capable of expecting a child mentally as a total person, beyond the concrete physical gesture of carrying it.

Various ways of containing

There are big differences in the way patients conceive of the concept of a container, and we can observe them developing it in the course of their analysis.

In fact, 'there are various containers, each with its own manner of containing: inert containers that do not interact with their passive contents; the containers which act on their contents; the containers that produce or create their contents. This leads us to the idea of a container that engenders a living content, which presupposes a primal scene and filiation' (D. Quinodoz 1992b: 629). That idea helps us to discover that, if we treat the creative containing function of the analyst as capable of engendering its contents, that is, the analytic process, we are brought closer and closer to the container–contained concept formulated by Bion (1962), the analyst's creative container capacity being expressed by the sexual encounter between container and contained. In fact, for the analytic process, as an engendered content, to come into being, the container must be a dynamic encounter of parents; it can then be symbolized as Bion has done, by sexual symbols, male and female, representing the container and the contained respectively.

When the analysand discovers the various shades of the means of containing, he no longer clings to the unequivocal image of the hollow, containing receptacle which sometimes refers to the female sex; in the many ways of containing he discovers the concept of multiple links that can bind the various components of the contained by internal cohesion; the contained then has an internal containing force and has less need for an external container. The containing organ can now be symbolized by an inner force of cohesion instead of by an external agency. This symbolization is important because the patient realizes that the penis can have a containing function in much the same way as the vagina or uterus and, moreover, that at the highest level the encounter of male and female is the best way of symbolizing the containing capacity.

It should be noted that the concept of the analyst-container, inasmuch as it implies creativity, is not based on the dual notion of the fabrication of a lifeless product, but is close to the triangular notion of procreation. The images involved reflect this situation clearly: even if the breast as a part object can evoke a dual relationship for the patient, the analyst sees it as a triangular relationship, the mother being unable to bear or to breastfeed a child unless the father has been involved. When an early relationship is relived in the transference, the analyst does not consider it a dual relationship, even if it seems to be so for the analysand, but an early triangular relationship, because the father is present in the reverie of the mother-analyst.

Psychic space also has a temporal dimension; integration of a traumatic experience into the patient's personal history

Why had Luc forgotten that crucial event (his mother talking to him about her attempted abortion) and not recalled it until this point in the analysis? Why had a split-off part of his ego been built round this event? In fact, when a patient is unable to remember an important scene he has experienced, it is often because it is too frightening to be included in his personal history. Either by isolating it or by denying it outright, he prevents the construction of links between that moment in his life, a source of so much anxiety, and the rest of his existence; it is as if he were trying to make sure that it cannot contaminate the rest of his life.

We can imagine that upon hearing about his mother's plan, Luc had felt such libidinal and aggressive stirrings that he had been frightened by the part of himself capable of producing these affects and impulses; he had accordingly tried to suppress them unconsciously. It was only during analysis that, with the help of the analyst, he dared to look at these inner forces, whereupon they appeared to him in a different and less frightening light.

It is not enough, in fact, to show the analysand the mechanism by which he turns his back on painful experiences: inasmuch as the conflict from which he defends himself is too frightening, his survival demands that he cling to his defence mechanism; if he absolutely must, he may be prepared to change it for a more adequate one. It is only when, in the course of his psychoanalysis, he has learned to modify his inner conflicts, his instinctual forces at work and his inner objects that he can discard a defence mechanism; in that case, what used to prove excessively frightening has become much less so, with the result that recourse to the old defences has become pointless. The integration by the analysand of memories of traumatic events into his personal history brings out the temporal dimension of psychic space.

4

Suction-related vertigo

Anxiety about being sucked up by the object

Suction-related vertigo may be considered the complement of vertigo related to being dropped. In fact, these two forms of vertigo correspond to two phantasies evoking complementary corporeal resonances: the intense anxiety about being dropped by a containing object which flies open and spills its content is the direct opposite of the anxiety about being kept prisoner for all time by a container that does not allow its content to escape.

This type of vertigo is very close to claustrophobia, the phobic fear of being kept in a closed space; the claustrophobic patient's panic is generally linked to the phantasy that he cannot get out of this space, and goes with physical symptoms commonly associated with fear, such as respiratory difficulties, palpitations or dizziness. For Melanie Klein, 'claustrophobia goes back to the fear of being shut up inside the mother's dangerous body' (1932: 329; 1946: 305).

Suction-related vertigo is sometimes mistaken for claustrophobia, but it goes much further; in fact, the symptom does not only appear when the patient finds himself in a closed place in which he might feel imprisoned; it appears every time he is in a situation reminding him of the phantasy of being sucked up by an enclosed object and kept imprisoned inside it. The situation varies from one analysand to the next; thus Lise said that she lost her balance when she went out skiing one day and came across a *ratrac*, a machine that levels out ski slopes: it reminded her irresistibly of the anxiety she had felt as a little girl about being sucked up by her mother's vacuum cleaner.

However, what struck me as most characteristic of this condition was that, for suction-related vertigo to appear in a patient susceptible to it, it is enough for him to have the feeling (without any apparent cause) that he is not free physically or psychically, that is, the phantasy of being held prisoner

45

by an internal object. On the couch, I have seen patients who, experiencing suction-related vertigo or talking to me about it, would violently kick and lash out at imaginary oppressors; others who had dizzy spells when suddenly feeling oppressed by the constraints of the analytic setting, or unable to tolerate the fundamental rule, which demands that the analysand tell the analyst whatever comes to his mind. This last group of patients sometimes gained the impression that I was standing behind them like an immense vacuum cleaner, watching them in readiness for swallowing them up, or like a siphon ready to suck them into myself never to let them go again. They tried to explain away the paralysis of their associative thoughts with such comments as: 'How could I possibly tell you everything that crosses my mind when my words are sucked into a prison in which they will be kept forever!' Quite often, too, it was through the feeling of losing their breath that these patients expressed the fear of losing their inner freedom, as if the object was about to swallow up their air.

For a patient to rid himself of this type of vertigo, he must be helped to verbalize his feelings in analysis, and then, little by little, to verbalize the phantasies associated with these feelings. Vertigo assumes the greater psychic meaning the more the analysand rediscovers phantasies that he has excluded from consciousness.

The analyst as a devouring mouth

Among my patients, Luc had the most anxiety-provoking manifestations of suction-related vertigo; when that happened he was close to delirium during analysis: on the couch, he felt that he was at the edge of an abyss about to turn into the mouth of a ferocious dog ready to swallow him up. In nothing so much as in the transformation of this phantasy did Luc evince that he was making progress in his analysis: the abyss, from being passive as it had been at first, assumed a lively will of its own filled with instinctual aggressive drive[1]. The extreme nature of what Luc was feeling helped me to a better understanding of the less lurid phantasies of other patients.

The reason why Luc felt that the mouth-analyst threatening to swallow him up was a void was that, in an unconscious aggressive phantasy, he imagined he had emptied me of all I might contain; this led him to phantasize that I was about to change into the mouth of an aggressive dog ready to swallow him up in revenge for having been emptied. In other words, I was holding him prisoner to recover what he had stolen from me or broken by emptying me.

The envy mechanisms I have mentioned in connection with Luc can also be encountered in female patients, who may phantasize that their mother wants to breathe into them what they imagine they have stolen from her.

46

The daughter then finds herself inextricably tied to her mother, in a relationship of two envious persons who threaten to take or recapture what they phantasize they have stolen from each other.

The associated fear is actually a 'retaliation' anxiety in the original meaning of the term *lex taliones*, because the analysand phantasizes that the analyst-mother, a castrator by suction, is about to apply the maxim 'An eye for an eye, a tooth for a tooth'. This form of anxiety is played out at the part-object level, which accounts for its intensity: in fact, the dog's mouth I was for Luc was an isolated object, not even attached to the animal; and Luc, in his associations, gave me to understand that what he phantasized he had stolen corresponded to a very regressive view of the contents of the maternal belly.

Babies carved or moulded by their mothers

To understand Luc's phantasy attacks on my womb, I must refer the reader to Melanie Klein's explanation of how the maternal womb is conceived as a confused and omnipotent cloaca, vaguely containing paternal penises, babies and faeces, and reminiscent of the interchangeability of the concepts of faeces, baby and penis mentioned by Freud (1917c). Luc gradually rediscovered certain phantasies relating to what for him were the highly intriguing and frightening contents of the all-engulfing maternal womb. For instance, he phantasized that it was by carving out penises in her belly that a mother makes babies; this reinforced his phantasy of the all-engulfing mother; another phantasy was that the mother's womb was a baker's oven where the mother moulds penises into babies and then bakes them, pushing forward those that are golden brown, and pushing back any that are overdone, the 'black pooh'. This takes us into the register of signal anxiety intended to prevent outbursts of the patient's oral and anal libido.

The vagina sucking in the penis and keeping it prisoner

Fragmented and global part objects

The phantasies mentioned so far bore mainly on the contents of the mother's womb and on fragmentary part objects. Suction-related vertigo often elicits other sexual phantasies which I consider even more anxiety-inducing, because they are based on global part objects. Clinical experience has led me to distinguish between *global* part objects and those I have called *fragmented*.

The breast, for example, may be a *global* part object if it represents the whole mother, all her functions being vested in the breast, the rest of her seemingly having the sole role of expressing her feeding function; when Luc, recumbent on the couch, voiced the phantasy of being nothing but a penis, that is, a global part object, he realized that he took for semen the viscous white liquid that sometimes seemed to invade his head and prevented him from thinking, so much so that his head ceased to be a head and assumed the functions of his penis.

On the other hand, the breast can also be a *fragmented* part object, in which case the child only considers the feeding side of the mother, the object of desire of his partial oral instinct, to the detriment of all the other maternal functions which he chooses to ignore; when Luc imagined a primal scene between fragmented part objects, it was coitus involving nothing but the encounter of a penis with a vagina, rather than of a father with a mother. Needless to say, these theoretical distinctions reflect two extreme poles of a tendency that we encounter only in its intermediate stages.

The partial nature of the object bestows a disturbing character on it, because it suggests that the object lacks intentionality and cannot be argued with and made to see reason. Anxiety is pronounced even in the case of fragmented part objects, which either bring out the value of one aspect of the object to the detriment of all the rest, or else juxtapose aspects of the object without synthesizing them; thus Marcelle Spira noted that fairy tales tend to dwell on the most disturbing characteristics of part objects: for instance, severed arms may carry torches to guide the lost traveller through the fairy's or the monster's mysterious castle.

However, I believe that anxiety is greater still in the case of global part objects, that is, when the entire object is reduced to one of its aspects or to one of its functions; this often happens with the sexual phantasies underlying suction-related vertigo: the analysand, prisoner of a mother identified with her swallowing vagina, feels that he is completely identified with the swallowed-up penis. What we have here is a particularly frightening primal scene, because it takes place between global part objects, the part being mistaken for the whole.

Male and female phantasies

An analysand suffering from suction-related vertigo told me that this condition corresponded to the sensation that the erection of his penis depended entirely on the vagina that sucked it in. He painted a picture of a frightening primal scene in which the mother was so powerful that the sucked-in penis ended up by merging with the vagina; the penis, reduced to a sucked-in surface, then adhered to the surface of the vagina, like a finger of a reversible glove that, if viewed from inside, was the vagina and, viewed from the outside, was the penis.

This phantasy is very frightening because, by closing the gap between the sexes, it does away with the difference, and hence with any possible relationship, between them. At the start, there are indeed two objects, but the absorption transforms them into a single and terrifying fused object. The frightening nature of that object springs from its paralysing ambiguity: its vagina-aspect and its penis-aspect blend into a single amalgam which, superseding the possibility of dialectical exchanges between the sexes, produces a feeling of paralysis. This paralysing anxiety can be found, for instance, in certain analysands who have a primitive phobic fear of snakes; that phobia can have different meanings, one of which corresponds to the primitive image of the snake that bites and swallows: an ambiguous snake penetrating and absorbing all at once and so conjuring up a confusion of the two sexes.

The phantasy of the penis being absorbed by the vagina is not confined to male patients. Janine Chasseguet-Smirgel has discussed *swallowing up* in connection with a claustrophobic female patient: 'To reach the Oedipus stage, she must identify herself with a castrating mother, that is, *swallow the father's penis up into her vagina*' (1964: 142). In suction-related vertigo, the female genitals, as the swallowers-up, are imagined to be an enclosed organ, a prison; they may be empty, but they have walls, and the patient is afraid of being imprisoned inside.

The phantasy of the penis being swallowed up by the vagina may lead the female patient to another frightening phantasy: that of being swallowed up by her own mother because the patient has identified herself with her father or rather with her father's penis as a global part object. Lise, whose fear (sometimes mixed with the wish) of being swallowed up by *ratracs* on the pistes, the machines I mentioned at the beginning of this chapter, remembered during her analysis the context in which, as a child, she became panic-stricken by the vacuum cleaner her mother was using: this happened at a time when the mother kept complaining about her husband to Lise and confided in her what she planned to do to keep him at home. Lise, who was then in an oedipal phase of adoring her father, defended herself against her ambivalent feelings by identification with her father, and dreaded being imprisoned by her mother as she imagined her father was about to be.

The phantasy that one's own thoughts might be sucked in by another's

Suction-related vertigo can also be experienced at the intellectual level. It is quite common for an analysand to mention that on occasion he experienced vertigo due to being sucked in by the thought of another person, which gave him the feeling of losing his critical faculties and of being unable to think anything except what the other put into his head.

This was the case with Rosa, a very talented analysand in whom the fear of being sucked up by her mother had taken the form of suction-related vertigo linked to her reading. As a small child, Rosa had learned to read aloud without difficulty, but she had had problems in grasping the underlying meaning of what she was reading out. As an adult, her diffi-culties continued: either she completely rejected the text she had read, or else she was totally absorbed by it, being able to repeat it or summarize it, but not to take a critical view of it. The text thus became the prison of Rosa's thought.

Here I shall not retrace the course of the analytic process by which Rosa came to feel that she was benefiting from the lack of free space between her parents and herself. All I wish to show is what a patient may express when suction-related vertigo abates and he succeeds in finding a corporeal repres-entation for what is going on inside him, that representation then serving him as a signpost when looking for a meaning in this type of vertigo and in changing the particulars of the underlying conflict.

One day Rosa turned up deeply distressed; at the end of the previous ses-sion, and too late to tell me about it, she had realized that I had misunderstood what she had said. Normally I took care to let Rosa know what I failed to understand in her remarks, to underline the differences between us. For the first time, Rosa now told me that she refused to be taken over by my thoughts and wished to uphold her own opinions against mine; but that seemed a tragedy to her. When, in the course of the current session, she came to realize gradually that there was no real drama, she began to sense the possible meaning for her of the vertigo related to the fear of being sucked up by someone else's thoughts; she then associated it with an experience trivial in itself but full of corporeal references: she had always been afraid, while skiing, of being dragged uphill on a T-bar because she felt she was being irresistibly sucked up by the person standing beside her, and relied on that person to keep her on the prepared tracks; it often ended in a fall. Recently, however, Rosa had come to feel, through some kind of internal corporeal revelation that it was not up to the other person to keep both of them on the tracks, but up to her to follow her own piste and to worry about her own balance, without however forgetting that two people were using the same T-bar. This representation of her suction-related vertigo appeared the moment her symptom began to make sense in the analysis and its manifestations became less acute. Rosa had discovered, in connection with an experience involving corporeal sensations, a representation of the vertigo repeated during analysis and invested with a symbolic meaning helping her to understand the analytic transference relationship. The analysand and I were sharing a T-bar, each trying to find his own equilibrium, each following his own tracks even while being linked and pursuing a single objective.

A withdrawal that makes sense in the counter-transference

During sessions in which Luc experienced states close to suction-related vertigo, I realized suddenly that I had withdrawn mentally: I caught myself thinking hard about something else. That sort of withdrawal was unusual enough for me to wonder if it might be connected with the analytic work on which my patient and I were jointly engaged, because, in that case, it was important that I came to understand its significance if I was to grasp what was happening between us. During a session with Luc in which this sort of withdrawal occurred, it became clear to me that what I had acted out in my counter-transference by mentally escaping from the session had at least two meanings.

The first meaning, that I must not allow myself to be sucked in by the analysand, was an attempt at personal safety by which I placed myself out of reach of Luc's unconscious need to imprison me; in fact, Luc's fusional monologue had the effect, unconscious on his part, of preventing me from thinking for myself and of draining me of my own thought; my response, unconscious to begin with, but becoming conscious when I thought about it, was to recover my own thoughts, in an attempt not to get sucked up by Luc's monologue. It was important for me to become conscious of that first unconscious reaction if I was to make use of it: as long as it remained unconscious, I acted out my withdrawal without being able to take advantage of it in my relationship with Luc.

In effect, Luc and I could only analyse his phantasy of emptying me if he was able to convey it to me in his own way; since he found it difficult to verbalize it, he communicated it by living it out in his sessions with me; but in order to allow himself to do that, it had to be harmless, that is, we would have to face his phantasy without my allowing it to become a reality. In short, for Luc to be able to express his phantasy of emptying me and for us to analyse it, I had to guard consciously against being emptied of my own thoughts.

The second meaning, accepting the projection of the analysand's need to escape, brought in my capacity for reverie as an analyst. I realized that my withdrawal from the session was partly the result of the projection into myself of Luc's need to get out of reach of the 'dog's mouth' of the session. In that session, Luc had been afraid that I might bite him with my interpretations and that I was keeping him prisoner, but he had felt it in too confused a way to become fully conscious of it and to verbalize it for me. He was like the very young child who does not know what to do with its alarming feelings and projects them into his mother so that she might de-dramatize them and allow them to be integrated.

I felt a need to escape, and that need corresponded in part to the projection into me of Luc's own need to escape; it would moreover be more correct to say that, at first, I actually withdrew at one point during the session before becoming conscious of my wish to escape and wondering about its significance. It was only subsequently that, paying heed to my counter-transference, I came to understand that my withdrawal from the session had a meaning; I could then bring it home to Luc that his own escape also had a meaning. After that, I was able to make use of my counter-transference instead of acting it out.

With analysands suffering from suction-related vertigo, as with those suffering from vertigo related to being dropped, the use the analyst makes of his counter-transference is put very severely to the test, because the patient makes considerable use of projective identification and of infraverbal means of communication; it is only as he extends his psychic space that he gains greater freedom to make use of verbalization and symbolism.

Note

1 I have used 'drive' as the translation of the German *Trieb*, retaining 'instinct' only in quotations from the *Standard Edition*.

5

Imprisonment/escape-related vertigo

Two active tendencies:
fleeing from the object and returning to it

Imprisonment/escape-related vertigo may be summed up as follows: the analysand who feels in his regressive part that the shelter-providing analyst keeps him imprisoned may have an urge to escape from the prison to breathe freely again; but once outside the prison he finds himself cut off from the object, which in his fusional mode of relating means facing the void or a fall; he accordingly seeks out the prison once more to escape from the void; but in that prison he is filled with just one idea, namely that of escaping. Now this alternating prison–escape process can go on for a long time and make the analysand feel dizzy.

One might be tempted to think that vertigo associated with the alternation of imprisonment and escape is simply the juxtaposition of the vertigo associated with the feeling of being dropped into the void by the object (vertigo related to being dropped), and the opposite type of vertigo, that of being kept prisoner by the object (suction-related vertigo). This is reminiscent of the inseparable alternation of claustrophobia and agoraphobia. The claustrophobic patient is afraid of staying in a closed space: he imagines that he is being kept prisoner in it; now, very often this self-same patient also suffers from agoraphobia: when he is out in the open he feels lost in the void, because he does not notice the presence of a whole network of connections between him and his surroundings, which would enable him to find out where he is. It is clear that the problem of claustrophobic and agoraphobic patients in relating to their surroundings often reflects the difficulties they have in structuring their psychic space and in relating to internal objects.

In fact, imprisonment/escape-related vertigo reflects an object relationship quite other than that which appears when there is a juxtaposition of vertigo related to being dropped and suction-related vertigo.

If an analysand juxtaposes vertigo related to being dropped and suction-related vertigo he finds himself, in his phantasies, either in prison or in the void; he cannot conceive of any other possibilities and moves straight from the one to the other. In imprisonment/escape-related vertigo, by contrast, the analysand does not immobilize himself inside a prison or the void, but moves between the two, actively fleeing the one to find the other. The more strongly he experiences this alternation of imprisonment and escape, the more he discovers the presence of a third possibility, one that is neither fusion with the object nor a void outside the object but a relationship with the object, presupposing a space in which links between him and the object can be established. This new space, allowing of movement and of uncertainty, opens the door to a mode of relating other than the fusional. As a result of the experience of actively moving to and from the prison–object, the analysand discovers the object-relational mode in which distinct objects are interconnected and no longer considered as prisons; in this new mode of relating the links between the analysand and the objects allow the preservation of the separate existence of each partner, instead of causing one of the partners to disappear, as happens in fusion or in the void.

Vertigo appears during the transition from the mode of fusional relationship to the object-relational mode, the latter not yet being sufficiently familiar and tested to be experienced without apprehension.

The emergence of a frontier zone

The mode of relating which passes on from fusion straight to the void, and which the analysand begins to be able to renounce during this transition, corresponds to what Melanie Klein has called the paranoid-schizoid position. Despite the giddy-making nature of the transition, the analysand somehow finds great relief in abandoning the fusional mode of relationship, which is extremely trying for him: in effect, while experiencing the juxta-position of being dropped and being imprisoned, the analysand might find his mood changing from one minute to the next without understanding why: one moment he is relatively happy, the next he feels desperate, abandoned or crushed.

We can imagine that, in the paranoid-schizoid position, the two moods clash, are juxtaposed, as if there were no way out and no shock absorber. The analysand's internal landscape looks like a flat world with two swivelling sides or faces: he finds himself on one or the other of these sides and while he is on it, the other is not only invisible but also unimaginable. If the analysand's mood is black, it cannot be mitigated by the mood characteristic of the other face; there is no space between the two in which he might store the memory of the other.

During the active coming-and-going into and out of the fusion corresponding to imprisonment/escape-related vertigo, the analysand gradually realizes that he does not pass on from fusion straight to the void. The new space that is beginning to take shape for him, even though it may well be no more than a no man's land at first, enables him to appreciate that he is not passing on from two fused persons to two unrelated persons, but from two fused persons to two distinct persons between whom there is a relational space and not a void. His inner world then seems voluminous, filled with connections and subtle nuances that allow him to proceed from one inner landscape to another without forgetting the first.

The patient discovers his active role

An active to-and-fro movement facilitating the construction of space

The reason why imprisonment/escape-related vertigo throws light on the analytic process is largely that it reveals a transitional state and helps the patient to discover new possibilities. He begins to feel that he has an active role to play in establishing relations with his objects, and that proves to be essential if, in his regressive part, he is to begin to conceive of the possible existence of space outside the fusion. The analysand has the feeling of *fleeing actively* from the object and no longer of *being dropped passively* by it as in vertigo related to being dropped; and of *returning actively* to the object instead of *being passively sucked up* by it as in suction-related vertigo. Thanks to this active coming-and going-into and out of his prison-refuge, he can slowly construct a three-dimensional *space* in the place of the *void*.

The omnipotence of the object and the idealization of the fusion diminish as soon as an analysand begins to realize that he has something to do with what happens to him; he is then confronted with all the multifarious feelings coexisting within him, with all his conflicts, with all his contradictory desires, which can lead him, with his analyst's help, to the symbolic discovery that his inner space has a volume infinitely greater than he ever imagined, and that he can allow for the coexistence in him of a whole complexity of the most varied affects.

Between anxiety about losing the ego by fusion and that of losing the object by defusion

That is why, when I gained the impression that an analysand found himself in the borderline zone between the fear of losing the object by defusion and the fear of losing his ego by defusing himself from it, I tried by my interpretations to help him enlarge that borderline zone, bringing out its complexity and richness so that he might discover a new solution: differentiation from the object, facilitating communication with it.

Let me take the case of patients who, feeling dizzy when faced with the problem of arriving at a satisfactory relationship with the analyst, make abusive remarks about the analysis. When their vertigo is due to the difficulty of maintaining their contradictory desires of fleeing from the object–prison and seeking refuge in it, their words, apparently designed to persuade the analyst to reject them, might hide a great longing for tenderness and also the need to be kept on in analysis. These analysands give me the impression of using their verbal barbs to keep me at bay, though these barbs also hide the opposite desire, namely to be fondled. They are like hedgehogs which must not be touched if you do not want to get hurt, but which surprise you because, if you get over that first impression and pick them up firmly, they do not prick you and even let you discover the downy and fragile belly which their spines protect. To one of these patients, I said: 'It's as if you liked me to hold you in my arms, close enough for you not to feel that I was about to drop you but not too close for you to feel imprisoned.' I thus tried, bearing the context in mind, to bring out the correspondence between the analysand's corporeal perceptions and his complementary and opposite psychic aspirations.

Discovery of the object-relational mode

The incessant exertions of the analysand who wears himself out reaching for the *one* and then dropping from the *one* into three-dimensional space mark progress over his previous immobility which idealized or denigrated fusion, because his efforts create the conditions for discovering the object–relational mode. This is an advance on agoraphobia and claustrophobia, two forms that vertigo can assume when the analysand realizes the danger entailed by fusion, yet has no alternative but to succumb to another danger, the void, because he still finds it hard to believe that he might take a third route, the object-relational, to communicate with a separate object.

I was struck by the story of a man who, having learned to hang-glide, gave voice to his discovery of space; his explanation seemed to be a symbolic hint of what the discovery of relational psychic space might be. He expressed his surprise in the following words: 'Before, when I stood on the peak of the Salève and looked at the Jura, there was a complete void between the two; rationally, I knew of course that there was air between them, but I had the feeling that on taking off from the Salève with my hang-glider I was about to fling myself into nothingness, into the void; but while actually flying, I could hear the voice of the teacher who had told me about space, and I began to feel and see that this particular void was full. The reason why I saw this space taking shape was that I felt the effects of what I was seeing: over there, on top of the lucerne field a column of air was rising, over there a lateral current might pull me a long way from the landing strip, and over there, against the mountain, there was much down draught and turbulence. I was not yet very familiar with that space, but I could rely on it and play with it.' We thus learn that the corporeal discovery of space involves the experience of being active in that space, of relating to the surrounding objects. My informant added: 'While I thought there was nothing between me and the Jura mountains, I could not tell if they were near or far – they were out of reach. When I felt the consistency of the space between us, it came within reach and I could gauge my distance from the mountains.' That space took shape, it was filled: criss-crossed by links between the objects and the active subject, allowing one not only to position oneself but also to reach the other – it was a 'carrying' space.

Envisaging an active role may lead to apprehension

A container that keeps and expels

The discovery of the space in which the analysand actively flees the object only to rejoin it again actively, enables him to take a fresh view of what he expects of the object's containing attitude. Analysands who go through periods of fusion-related vertigo, of vertigo related to being dropped, or of suction-related vertigo, often have a very rudimentary understanding of the container they tend to idealize. In their eyes, the 'ideal' container is ever-present; the 'good' analyst is one who never goes on vacation and who extends the sessions for the analysand's convenience; they, furthermore, imagine that the 'good' analysand wants each session to go on for ever and hopes that the analysis will never to come to an end.

'For example, one of my analysands had the fantasy that if a pregnant woman contained her baby with love, she would wish to keep it for ever, and the midwife would have to rip it away from her by force. This analysand was very surprised to discover during analysis that a mother who contains her baby puts just as much energy into carrying it within her as she does into expelling it actively when the time comes' (D. Quinodoz 1992b: 630). In short, he discovered that a good container is capable of keeping the contained object *in* as well as of pushing it *out*. 'Taken separately, each term of the container function – keeping "inside" and pushing "outside", may assume an aggressive, death-dealing character. In the former case it is asphyxiation and in the latter, rejection, as well as the impossibility of estab-

57

lishing a continuous object or object relation. It is the synthesis of the two terms that allows the container to function properly' (*ibid*.).

Active participation in the act of being expelled

The discovery of the container–contained interaction enabled this analysand to become aware not only of the active role of the container during expulsion, but also of the active role of the contained. It proved a shock to him when he realized that it was not the mother alone who pushes the baby out, but that the baby itself contributes to its own expulsion: it does what it has to do to come out and to be born. Such realizations by the analysand are very important when he envisages the end of a session or the end of his analysis. The analysand is sometimes surprised to discover that much as the 'good analyst' is not the one who keeps his patients on for good, so the 'good analysand' can want a session to come to an end and the analysis to terminate.

The comforts of passivity

Awareness of the active part played by the ego in the construction of the object and the relationship is not devoid of anxiety for the analysand, inasmuch as it increases his responsibility and hence his guilt. In a way, being at the mercy of the object that drops him or sucks him up gives the analysand some comfort: everything is the object's 'fault', so that he, the analysand, is never to blame. It is remarkable that, at the beginning of their analysis, many patients stress the fact, sometimes with a degree of pleasure, that they are the victims of their nearest and dearest: according to them, their parents, their marriage partners or their children are wholly responsible for their present difficulties. If the analyst tries to mitigate the thrust of that accusation, he is likely to be rebuffed by the patient with: 'Surely you are not trying to make excuses for them!' As the analysis progresses, these patients come gradually to appreciate the importance of their active participation, and to go less and less in search of a scapegoat. They become increasingly interested in their own motives and those of others.

6

Vertigo due to attraction to the void: the emergence of internal space

The irresistible attraction of the void: the feeling of external void as projection of the feeling of internal void

Vertigo due to attraction to the void, which is very common, assumes two forms. In the more active one, the patient says: 'I have an overwhelming desire to throw myself into the void'; he may tell you, for instance, how he has to keep away from the edge of the balcony, for although he has no conscious desire to kill himself, he nevertheless has an urge to jump into the void. The second form is more passive, the patient saying: 'I am irresistibly drawn to the void', and he will also avoid getting close to windows or to the edge of a precipice, because everything seems unsteady and a whirlwind seems about to suck him up, not in order to imprison him as in suction-related vertigo, but to make him disappear.

This vertigo in its two forms introduces excorporation as well as projection mechanisms. The attracting external void often turns out to be a projection of the patient's feeling that he has an inner void. He has different ways of feeling anxious about, and fascinated by, the external void, depending on what he projects into it; moreover, depending on his projections, this attractive *outside* changes: it may be felt to be an unfathomable external void, but equally well a relational space filled with riches. Between these two feelings there can be a whole range of intermediate stages. The anxiety about being irresistibly attracted to this void or to this space can be associated with various representations invested with bodily references.

In addition to differing in that they may be active or passive, the two forms of vertigo due to attraction to the void can also be distinguished by the phantasies underlying them, namely phantasies about fragmented or global part objects.

59

*The active form: I feel like throwing myself into a void,
which is already a space*

The phantasies accompanying the active form of vertigo due to attraction to the void most commonly involve fragmented part objects.

When analysands begin to realize that they themselves and the objects from which they try to distinguish themselves are not necessarily divided by a void but by a relational space, their response is often highly ambiguous. To them, this space is still the *void* towards which they can adopt a passive attitude, but already a *space* in which they have an active part to play; they can then grow fascinated with this peculiar void-space to the point of developing an overwhelming desire to throw themselves into this *intermediate* structure, as if they had a pressing need to recover something in it. This desire to fling oneself into a fascinating void-space is something quite other than allowing oneself to be sucked up by the object, and also differs from the impulse to flee from, or seek out, the object; what worries and fascinates patients presenting vertigo due to attraction to the void is the desire to discover relational psychic space criss-crossed with links between objects. What we have here is an internal psychic space which these patients hope to discover unconsciously by means of their perception of external space. The analysis of this type of vertigo reflects the mixture of anxiety about the void and the hope of discovering that it is not really a void but an inhabited, relational space. That phase can be very trying for the analyst because there is a marked risk that the analysand may start to act out. That happened with Luc, who felt an irresistible desire to throw himself into the void and more particularly through the window.

For analysands susceptible to this form of vertigo, the fascinating void-space is paradoxically both *empty* and *filled*, and becomes the representation of *outside* and *inside* at one and the same time.

**This void-space becomes an external space filled with matter when the
patient packs it with what he cannot bear to keep inside himself**

In fact, when a patient shifts all responsibility onto the object, ascribing a purely passive role to himself, it is often because he is frightened by the force of his instincts and does everything in his power to avoid blame. The obvious reason why he deploys these regressive defence mechanisms in a split-off part of his ego is that he is trying unconsciously to protect the rest of his ego from the violence of his drives. When the analysand begins to rediscover the active part he has to play in his object relationship, he also rediscovers the panic caused by the violence of his drives. Having recovered his active part in the relationship, he is once again confronted with the danger that caused him to abandon it in the first place.

If the patient no longer wishes to resort to this old defence mechanism and to revert to passivity, he may have recourse to a projective defence mechanism which is a preliminary to vertigo related to attraction to the void: he will unconsciously project *outside* himself all those needs, desires and affects that he believes pose a threat to him. He then behaves as if they did not belong to him, and hence shelves his responsibility for them. He projects them to the *outside* into the void-space they thus fill in his phantasy.

Thus Luc, who was terribly afraid of his own violence and of his aggressive sexual drives would, at such moments, view his aggression in the shape of a hand detached from his own person and hence capable of battering someone to death without involving him, or again in the form of a raping penis for which he was not responsible, because it too was detached from him. Even without using so extreme a case as Luc's, we are familiar with such expressions by our patients as: 'Rage took hold of me', 'My eyes played me a trick', 'My memory is at fault', 'It was stronger than me', which reflect the feeling that this rage, these eyes, this memory, are not characteristic of the patient himself, but that he is their passive victim. In a way, the patients get rid of their impulses by disowning them. We see the beginnings of the anxiety reflected in vertigo: the patient who projects into the void-space those parts of himself he disapproves of also realizes that he is impoverishing himself bit by bit: he may come to feel that he runs the risk of destroying himself by flinging all of himself into the void, much as he might throw the baby away with the bath water.

We might note that this defence mechanism is often used by elderly patients who find it hard to accept that they are getting on in years; they 'give the impression of detaching from themselves, in their phantasies, aspects of their personality from which they would like to dissociate themselves: they refer to a part of their body, or to one of their psychic functions such as their memory, or to their advanced age, as if these were no longer part of their personality . . . In the extreme case, age itself becomes an external excuse and, detached from the rest of the self, is held responsible by the patient for what he does not like in himself: "It's my age that's the trouble!" Advanced age thus expelled by the organizing ego helps to preserve an ideal image of oneself. Nevertheless, all such expulsions from the self are so many forms of impoverishment' (D. Quinodoz 1991a: 28). Now we know that many elderly people succumb to vertigo and can have frequent falls.

This void-space is empty when it is the projection of the patient's inner void

The analysand projecting his needs or affects outside himself may feel momentarily relieved of his responsibilities, but this often leaves him with an intolerable internal void; by pushing out what he does not like in himself, he has created a feeling of a frightening internal void, so much so that he can be led unconsciously to project this intolerable feeling on to the outside as well. The internal void thus becomes an external void: the patient feels the void no longer inside but outside himself. This feeling of an internal void projected to the outside then becomes combined with the analysand's other projections, with the needs and desires he has unconsciously expelled, creating an external void-space filled with positive and negative projections, simultaneously empty–full and inside–out.

Excorporation, a precursor of projection

In attempting to show what this filled-yet-empty space may mean to the analysand, I find it useful to refer to a transitional psychic mechanism which, I think, is close to what André Green has called excorporation – the precursor of projection. 'Excorporation, primary expulsion, involves the furthermost possible centrifugal projection. Where to? Everywhere and nowhere. What is projected is not localized in any particular spot; it infiltrates ambient space, lending it the diffuse affective tonality characteristic of persecutory experience' (Green 1971: 204). This all-or-nothing part may be felt as an external void by some analysands, who thus try to give it a first name; this void may well be a way of saying that while it is not something *inside*, there certainly is no *space outside* as yet. Green uses the following striking formulation: 'The outside is then "outside of" or "out of there" – out of here, demons! Get out of my body!' (*ibid.*: 200). We can now distinguish projection from excorporation more clearly: 'In my opinion, projection proper only exists when an object can receive what has been excorporated. In that case there emerges a *projective plane* that receives and collects what has been projected' (*ibid.*: 200). Aware that when I use the word 'void' I am echoing the patient who tries to name the indefinable, I would say that, at its limit, excorporation operates in the void and projection in a space or object.

The danger of acting out

Here I am not referring to the type of acting-out by which the patient fulfils his desire to fling himself into the void, but to the kind of acting-out by which he satisfies the drives he had tried to get rid of unconsciously by excorporation. In fact, during this period dominated by projection mechanisms, the analysand runs a considerable risk of unconsciously acting out the drives from which he had tried to break free. The analysand is unconsciously ruled by his drives, even if he acts as if his drives did not belong to him. The drives act, so to speak, independently, having ceased to be linked to the ego, which might try to harmonize them with the rest of the personality. To take a particular case: I felt worried that Luc might act out the violence he did not seem to recognize as his own and that he consequently did not control, turning it against me during his sessions with me.

Throwing oneself into the void to recover what has been projected into it

In the course of their analysis, patients begin to realize that loved objects can be criticized as well as appreciated, which corresponds to the depressive position as described by Melanie Klein. They become kinder not only to loved objects but also to themselves, that is, they grow more tolerant of, and hang on to, those aspects of themselves that they do not appreciate. They no longer need to disown them to love themselves: they can love themselves, as they can love the object, for better or for worse. This does not mean that they love their faults or the object's; on the contrary, the more they love themselves or the object, the more critical they are of their faults and the more they try to correct them, even while tolerating their presence. They put up with the fact that they or the object have objectionable sides, because they have gained a rounded view of a total person made up of a multitude of facets combining and lending colour to one another. They are no longer obsessed with the bad side of the personality that struck them before as threatening to contaminate the whole. Instead they have grown brave enough to consider as part of themselves even the internal void they have created with their expulsions; henceforth they are able to try amelioration instead of expulsion.

It is then that they may feel like flinging themselves into the void–space in order to recover and to reintegrate what they have expelled. They become drawn into an ambivalent process by this external void–cum–space filled with matter, the exteriorization of the internal void–cum–space filled with matter. This fascination develops as a pendant to the construction of what they discover to be an *internal space* capable of containing, in the dynamic sense of the word, their own needs, desires, affects, and thoughts and also the internal objects, even those they criticize.

Vertigo related to attraction to the void marks another transition in analysis; when the patient no longer feels an imperious need in the regressive part of himself to project 'outside', he no longer 'empties' himself: an internal psychic space is being created.

The passive form of vertigo related to attraction to the void: I am sucked up by the void

This form of vertigo is often accompanied by the unconscious phantasy that the *unfathomable* external void is like a *bottomless* maternal belly threatening to swallow up the father's penis. Sometimes this immense belly is imagined in a more precise fashion as a vagina, sometimes also as a womb, but in any case the idea of the lack of a bottom remains, because that is the characteristic feature of vertigo related to attraction to the void and what chiefly distinguishes it from suction-related vertigo. In the first case the analysand feels anxious about being drawn into a bottomless void in which he will disappear, whereas in suction-related vertigo he has the feeling of being sucked up by a closed object that will keep him imprisoned.

I might add that women patients can identify themselves with the unfathomable maternal belly which attracts, but that they can also identify themselves with the paternal penis that is being attracted. In their phantasies, my male analysands were mainly identified with the paternal penis.

Male analysands

This phantasy of the penis being attracted by the void may be found in male patients, who thus express the ambiguous and anxious relationship they maintain with the female sex. A case in point was one of my patients who became dizzy when, looking at the sky or at a very high ceiling, he felt as if he were being sucked up; he experienced a similar kind of vertigo when, going up in an aeroplane, he had the impression that the sky was about to swallow the aeroplane up; this patient became aware of his phantasy that the external void attracting him felt like an omnipotent, unfathomable female womb threatening to suck him in completely, and in which he might disappear.

We saw that Luc, in his suction-related vertigo, sometimes had a very similar phantasy: he phantasized that the analyst lurked behind him like a dog's mouth ready to swallow him up whole; that mouth was to him the image of a devouring and aspirating maternal belly. However there was one characteristic difference which I mentioned earlier: in the phantasy associated with vertigo due to attraction to the void the maternal womb is imagined as a diffuse void, without any shape and above all without a bottom, and as one into which the analysand is in danger of disappearing; whereas in suction-related vertigo, Luc imagined the maternal womb as a precise object having a shape and a bottom – a dog's mouth about to swallow him up and keep him prisoner in an enclosed cavity. We find the same difference in patients who have vertigo related to being sucked into a siphon (say, the plughole in the bath or the hole at the bottom of a lavatory bowl): in some of these patients their vertigo reflects the anxiety of being imprisoned or remaining stuck in the drain or tank; in others it reflects the fear of disappearing into the void.

Female analysands

When the phantasy of the penis being sucked in by the womb appears in a female patient, the projection of the womb into the external void is combined with a return of aggression against the analysand herself: her womb (identified with that of the mother) sucking in the paternal penis is projected outside in such a way that the exterior is felt to be an immense bottomless womb while the patient feels completely identified with the sucked-in paternal penis.

This phantasy has been described by Janine Chasseguet-Smirgel in connection with one of her patients, Anne, who had impulses to fling herself into the river or into the void (1964: 140). During analysis, this patient remembered that her father nearly drowned when swept away by a bottomless whirlpool, and she produced the following association: 'I had the picture of a penis being sucked in by a vagina' (*ibid.*: 142). Chasseguet-Smirgel adds: 'Everything happened . . . as if parental coitus was to Anne the aggressive incorporation by the mother of the father's penis . . . (the father swallowed up in the whirlpool). To reach the oedipal stage she would have had to identify herself with the castrating mother, that is, *swallow up the paternal penis into her vagina*' (*ibid.*: 142). But in her vertigo, Anne did not feel anxious about *swallowing* but about *being swallowed*, which Chasseguet-Smirgel explains as follows: 'Due to her guilt feelings, Anne lives out the oedipal genital impulse in her phantasies ('swallowing up' the father's penis as her mother does), but *turns the aggression against* herself, her entire body being identified with the paternal penis, while her destroying vagina is projected into the outer world experienced as a cavity into which she disappears. *This means that content and container have been inverted. She herself becomes the content which disappears in the container*' (*ibid.*: 142). The most primitive phantasy expressing this fact directly is the following: 'I am the hole into which my father (his penis) is swallowed up' (*ibid.*: 142).

I stress that it is a characteristic of vertigo due to attraction to the void that the female patient feels she is a hole, which implies the absence of a bottom and in a sense of a shape; her reaction would have been quite different had she imagined herself as a cavity or a hollow organ. In that case she would have had phantasies corresponding to suction-related vertigo.

The phantasy of passive vertigo related to attraction to the void generally involves global part objects

This phantasy on the part of patients, male or female, who feel absorbed by the unfathomable external void does not, in my opinion, occur at the genital level, even though a penis and a vagina are involved; it often concerns global part objects. Chasseguet-Smirgel has put it most perceptively as follows: 'The "genital" level of these phobias does not preclude deep alterations of the Ego, guilt about the relationship with the idealized father, often resulting in . . . numerous and grave early conflicts with the first object' (*ibid.*: 143). Clearly it is not because a phantasy involves a penis and a vagina that it must be placed at the genital level; for that to happen, these two terms would have to be used with reference to total persons and in the context of a synthesis of partial drives. That is not the case here.

Projecting a hole into the void, or projecting a hollow organ into space?

The evolution of the formulations used by male and female analysands demonstrates how this type of vertigo can progress from (a) an almost uncontrollable vertiginous impulse to (b) a form of vertigo that begins to make sense and to become tolerable, or even to disappear.

In the first case, the patient is attracted by a bottomless void, felt to be a female sex organ represented by a hole, that is, by an orifice opening onto nothingness, a shapeless and bottomless void that cannot hold a content and take care of it, but can only make it disappear. In the second case, the patient is attracted to organized space experienced as a female genital represented by a hollow organ, capable of holding its contents and taking care of them. The analysand feels that a space is taking shape outside as well as inside himself; there is no longer a void. Between these two extreme representations there is naturally room for a whole gamut of subtle differences.

The emergence of inner space: its repercussions

The analysis of vertigo related to attraction to the void in its active or passive form, enabling us to retrace the path from the feeling of an outer void to the feeling of an inner void, involves a growing awareness of inner space and the wish to get to know it. That awareness has innumerable repercussions at the object-relational level; here I shall merely mention a few.

The ego's organizing activity

The discovery of this inner space goes hand in hand with that of the *ego's organizing activity*; when that happens analysands often have dreams of the following type: they are fleeing in a panic from terrifying and savage wild beasts, but suddenly feel that they have the courage to face them, stop fleeing, turn round and, looking at them closely, come to realize that the animals are not all that savage, and that they could, in fact, tame them. Analysands may come up with numerous variations of this type of dream, but nearly all these dreams have a common denominator: the dream implementation of the unconscious desire no longer to flee from one's own libidinal and aggressive impulses, from one's needs and desires. These drives had previously been considered dangerous and had accordingly been pushed outside, like wild beasts that did not belong to the analysand. However, once an analysand dares to face them instead of fleeing from them, these drives turn out to be much less frightening; the analysand can retrieve and reintegrate them as his own: these two reactions reinforce each other, because when these forces are taken over by the organizing power of the ego, they become more governable and hence less frightening; now, the less frightening they are the less difficult is their reintegration.

It was after the interpretation of that type of dream that Luc was able to speak to me openly about his impulse to rape me, which had previously made him freeze with terror, and which he had expelled like some wild beast: it became controllable as soon as he dared to look upon it as his own. Luc expressed his phantasies as follows: 'Before, my penis was sort of detached from me and I was afraid of the mad things it might do without my being able to stop it; now I feel that it is linked to my head and to my heart, that it belongs to me, and I no longer fear that it might act without the consent of the whole of myself.' In my counter-transference, I was no longer afraid that Luc might decide to act out his phantasy during the sessions.

Modification of dependence on the object

The mobility of the object may cause vertigo

The discovery of the ego's organizing activity, entailing that of its active participation in the construction of the characteristics of the object and of relational space, change the subject's dependence on the object.

Thus, one of my patients realized that, during some sessions when he lay frozen on the couch 'like a stone effigy', he was bound to be 'heavier to bear', and hence more easily dropped by me, than he was in other sessions when his lively participation made him 'light to bear'. He evoked the picture of a *father* who finds it hard to carry his limp child, but easy to carry the same child when 'it holds on'. The analysand thus realized that my character as a 'dropping' analyst might depend on him, the analysand. In a general way, he realized that the analyst's attitude might partly be caused by that of the analysand, but also that the character of the object as it appeared to the analysand depends on phantasies he projects into it: in particular, the object might seem to be terrifying because of terror phantasies projected into it. Luc, for instance, at that time, was acting very aggressively towards me because he felt that I had forbidden him to go on professional tours. But he then realized that I had, in fact, never forbidden him to do anything, and that it was his own reluctance to grow up that led him, in the transference, to consider me as a parent who kept him under her thumb.

In fact, what the patient discovers when he takes cognizance of psychic space is the changing aspect of the object. Awareness of the shifting character of the object, never fully achieved in psychoanalysis, assumes a puzzling character for those who would like to feel reassured that they can *grasp* it firmly; they might easily gain the impression that nothing is stable and that the object always escapes those who believe they have grasped it. Anyone wondering about the object can succumb to vertigo like the walker who stumbles while moving ahead and wondering about his position at that very moment; sometimes it is very hard indeed to realize that dynamic equilibrium is a concatenation of unstable positions.

The mobility of the object may be a factor in psychic equilibrium

The mobility of the object capable of causing vertigo nevertheless constitutes one of the attractions of the object, because, being perpetually created, the object never ceases to surprise us. In fact, some analysands who, at the beginning of their analysis, believe that past external reality is immutable, tend to hold it solely responsible for their present difficulties: 'I have had this trauma in the past; I can do nothing about it; how can I possibly make it go away?' or 'There is nothing to be done about it any more. My parents are dead, they can no longer change!'

To these analysands the realization that the internal object keeps developing constitutes a turning point in their analysis. They come to appreciate with surprise that their psychic reality develops during analysis and that it then changes their perception of external reality, just like that of their internal reality. They can now see internal and external objects, present or past, in a fresh light, bring out previously unnoticed aspects of the object, elicit fresh memories and fresh associations that, in turn, will give rise to phantasies and desires entailing a constant development of internal objects in con-tinuous animation. They discover that even if the external objects belong to the past and have reached the end of their own destiny, the internal objects corresponding to these external objects continue to develop and hence cause the analysand's object relations and view of their external objects to develop. They will then be surprised to see their parents in a light they had never suspected: 'I never saw that side of my father (long since dead), and never realized what he actually said to me at the time!' This patient discov-ered her father's organizational qualities, when all she had remembered before was feeling critical of him; moreover she realized, by unconscious identification with him, that she had the same organizational skills.

In short, these patients have discovered the permanence of the object (and of the subject) despite its (their) development. 'The object in psychoanaly-sis is a continuous psychic creation which the ego produces in a constant toing and froing between external reality and psychic reality, each modify-ing the other . . . The object, as well as the ego, thus find themselves at the meeting point of the continuous and the discontinuous, the ego and the object changing perpetually even while preserving their permanent identity' (D. Quinodoz 1989a: 1142). If he is no longer to suffer from vertigo, the patient must feel that, in his psychic space, there is room for an encounter between the continuity and the discontinuity of the object. The continuity ensures permanence and helps to avoid anxiety, while the discontinuity prevents monotony, because a person all of whose aspects can never be known never ceases to be a mystery.

The enigmatic character of the object

In effect, this de-idealization of the object which no longer seems to be omnipotent demonstrates the enigmatic character of the latter and makes it more interesting. The analysand instead of accusing the object of not being completely reliable feels the desire to get to know it and, in particular, to understand the reason for what seemed to be so many faults. Luc, for exam-ple, tried to imagine the conditions under which his mother had felt the urge to have an abortion and phantasized a whole gamut of different feelings a pregnant woman might have in his mother's circumstances: it was as if a flat earth had opened and filled up. Luc translated this impression to me by saying: 'Outside it is no longer the void, but space, and space is full of things and people worth getting to know.' Donald Meltzer has shown how 'the thirst for knowledge, the wish to know rather than to possess the object of desire makes it possible to give the object its freedom' (1986: 14).

Permitted secondary curiosity

Seeing or knowing?

Becoming aware of internal space, which makes possible the expression at a new psychic level of what was previously acted out, transforms the analysand's attitude to curiosity and particularly to sexual curiosity. In fact, when everything happens as if one had to *act* to satisfy one's curiosity, curiosity is imbued with guilt or squarely repressed. The infant might imagine that in order to *know* what is in his mummy's belly, he would have to open it up and *look* inside. But often he prefers not to *be naughty*, or hurt somebody, even though aggressive wishes may unconsciously coexist with libidinal desires in him; in that case what can he do if he is not to abandon his curiosity? He can, for instance, try to disembowel his doll or his teddy bear instead of his mother, but the result is disappointing as long as he is looking for a concrete answer to his question; even if he were to repeat the operation several times, he will fail to find in the doll's belly what he hoped to find in his mother's. One analysand recalled her disappointment when her father, taking her at her word, had the doll X-rayed in order to prevent aggressive attempts to open its belly; the rods and springs the analysand saw on the X-ray picture did nothing to satisfy her curiosity.

The child can defer looking for the answers, sometimes giving good reasons for doing so, for instance by declaring: 'Later on I shall become a surgeon and then I shall see what goes on inside the belly'; others come up with sheer phantasies: 'When I grow up I shall have an eye at the end of my penis and it will look to see what it's like inside mummy's belly.' The main thing is that in all these examples priority is given to *seeing* concretely, which is tantamount to giving priority to the incestuous act. Now that act, when it involves seeing something that is *inside*, can be accompanied by a sadistic wish to open, to attack, and to destroy in order to look.

All these solutions can normally be conceived by a child who has not yet discovered an adequate level of symbolization and who believes that he must act concretely in order to know. It sometimes happens that an adult patient will retain, in a regressive part of himself, this attitude to curiosity, which inhibits it and invests it with a punishable character, while the rest of his personality has developed quite normally, without his even being aware of that attitude.

The case of Marc: even looking was dangerous

Marc was a very gifted patient, but his social and professional life was thwarted by an intellectual inhibition, which I felt was mainly an inhibition

70

of curiosity. Marc would feel faint and succumb to vertigo whenever he had to show his desire for knowledge in his professional life. Now Marc worked in a research department, and that caused him many conflicts. If his superiors ordered Marc to do a particular piece of research, Marc would do it, but inhibit every initiative of his own, which quickly put an end to his professional hopes.

Marc was sometimes attacked by feelings of faintness and vertigo on the couch, especially when he enumerated what he was seeing in front of him: in fact, he kept his eyes shut and what he then thought he was seeing looked as if it had been projected onto a cinema screen. These were bizarre objects that he could not connect and that he did not try to invest with any meaning. In short, during these sessions he did not dare to watch what came into his mind, look closely at his internal world projected onto an imaginary screen. I interpreted his inhibition against looking by associating it in particular with his inhibition about finding things out for himself and with his aggression. Marc behaved as if he could not possibly see me, his analyst-father-cum-mother in the transference, as anything but an external object, and hence failed to turn me into an internal object; he could only look at me on a screen before him instead of trying to get to know me emotionally. In general terms, his desire to understand the primal scene could only be projected onto an external stage (the screen) riddled with prohibitions (because he was unable to organize what he saw).

Marc then had a dream: he saw a large snake in a round bowl. A smaller snake, with bright eyes, also slithered about in the bowl. Marc, horrified, smashed the head of the smaller snake. When he recounted this dream to me, Marc not only felt that he had crushed the head of the small snake, but he also identified himself with it. His associations made it clear that this dream was the realization of two antagonistic unconscious desires: on the one hand, *the wish to know the primal scene and to participate in it*: by slithering about in the bowl, the small snake fulfilled his desire to see, eyes burning with curiosity, what the big snake, the paternal part object, was doing inside the bowl (a female part object). On the other hand, the opposite desire, namely *to prevent the fulfilment of his desire to give free rein to his curiosity and to participate in the primal scene*: by crushing the head of the smaller snake, Marc avoided – through preventive self-castration – the fulfilment of the first desire and the punishment it might have entailed. The dream thus provided a representation of the conflict, while expressing it in a regressive context of part objects.

In his dream, Marc had expressed the way in which his horror at the wish of the small snake to look at the primal scene was linked to the demand that the small snake must not be allowed to understand the primal scene with its head (and so he crushed its head). In fact, this is precisely what Marc was doing during analysis as well: in the analytic session, he crushed his own head; he banned the use of his own thought (his head) in trying to discover what was happening inside him; and he dared to use his eyes only to look at the screen outside; but even then he used them with restrictions, not allowing himself to link what he was seeing with his thoughts and phantasies, and hence not fitting it into a psychic structure. The dream and its interpretations provided Marc with enough material to gain some inkling of what was happening in his psyche; the more he used his head during the sessions, the more the vertigo and the faintness receded.

Coming to grips with the invisible

When an analysand such as Marc discovers that psychic activity also has a penetrating function making it possible to reach for the invisible, he becomes open to permissible secondary curiosity. Not only does he discover that when acting-out is forbidden, phantasy can be given free rein, he also discovers that everyone has the right to his own phantasies about the object. This happened to Marc, whose professional life took off when permissible secondary curiosity, consisting of phantasies about what he knew of me, his analyst-mother in the transference, replaced the sadistic incestuous curiosity which he felt was a punishable act.

In this connection, it may be worth noting that sex education classes for children may sometimes seem disappointing to the teachers because some children, obviously keen to know more, take little interest in the lessons, ask few questions and sometimes even demand to be told again what the teacher has just explained, as if they had understood nothing. These classes often provide good scientific and rational explanations, but children also need to imagine their own phantasies about what they have picked up about sexuality; phantasies of which they are not necessarily conscious but which, though they cannot express them, they feel vaguely to be reprehensible, an attitude that stands in the way of the acquisition of broader knowledge.

Psychic space combines with time: it does not exist outside its creator

In the course of his analysis, Luc was surprised to discover that he could bring me material during the session that had originated outside the session, and that conversely he could phantasize about my extra-analytic activities. He no longer had the feeling that he had to immobilize me in my consulting room between sessions, as he had done when he still believed that he ceased to exist for me outside. The splitting was no longer so pronounced and Luc expressed this by saying: 'Previously, I used to jump from session to session as one might from island to island; now there is no longer a void

between the islands; there is the sea and I can swim in it.' This was a colour-
ful way of saying that in the long run, the interval (time) between the
moments when we met contained a relational space and was no longer a void;
in this relational space which 'carried' us we could create associations; that
space was well worth discovering and we could enjoy it.

The 'sea' of which Luc spoke as an image of psychic space is a carrying
space for those who can swim. For those who cannot, it certainly is no void
either, but it does not carry them, it does not support human life. For
mental space to become a carrying space, the patient must be capable of
holding himself up; depending on our standpoint we can say that without
that *buoyancy* the patient will drown in the sea, or suffer separation anxiety
in even the most sympathetic surroundings. We need carrying space as well
as buoyancy. The two are complementary. We have seen several times, when
speaking of the mother's capacity for reverie, that it is by introjecting, thanks
to the transference, an analyst capable of lending meaning to his anxiety, that
the analysand discovers his own capacity for investing his anxiety with
meaning.

73

7

Expansion-related vertigo

Anxiety about expanding into a world without limits

Expansion-related vertigo occurs in analysands who realize that they keep puffing themselves up as if they needed this continuous expansion to feel that they are alive. They give one the impression that they will allow nothing to stand in the way of that continuous expansion. Actually, they have difficulties in determining the boundary between their ego and the object, and they begin to present vertigo the moment they realize that they have a need to get close to the limits of the object if they are to discover those of their ego, lest their ego spread by a form of expansion that robs it of shape and consistency.

I reserve a special place to expansion-related vertigo because it cropped up in peculiar and unexpected ways during the analysis of several patients who did not usually present vertigo. All had a narcissistic problem, and their vertigo always appeared in a similar transference context, just as if it were a signpost in the analysis of narcissistic patients. Now Luc, who presented all the other forms of vertigo in the course of his analysis, did not have expansion-related vertigo. For that reason, I have decided to dwell at some length on clinical vignettes drawn from the analysis of two other patients.

Testing the limits of the object to discover one's own

The narcissistic analysand subject to expansion-related vertigo generally has the impression that objects exist for his sake, and quite often he even feels that he is an altruist, or in any case has the ambition to be one; but in fact he does not consider objects as original persons living independent lives and hence interesting to know for their own sake; these objects interest him

74

above all inasmuch as they facilitate a better definition of himself; in short, they are the extension of his own ego. For example, one analysand lived in apparent harmony with his wife, but only because she was *his* spouse and because his married status was important in the definition of his image; he had children whom he expected to be appreciative of him; he took an interest in his colleagues, friends or lovers for just as long as they had interests that blended with his own and kept strictly within the bounds he had set them; the moment they started to ask something for themselves, be it time or active assistance, he stopped seeing or considering them.

In the course of his analysis, this type of analysand sometimes becomes aware that, as a result of this attitude, he has emptied his inner life of its objects. The realization that his life is *empty* can then go hand in hand with an attack of vertigo, because the impression that there is an absence of objects entails a feeling of ego loss due to the expansion of the ego into a world bereft of objects and hence unable to set the ego any limits. The analysand looks anxiously for the limits of an object against which he might come up in the attempt to discover his own limits and to feel that he exists.

These patients whose ego is apparently hypertrophied often prove to be very brilliant; they often seem very sure of themselves and are crushing to others; or their attitude may elicit an apparently paradoxical response from their family circle; far from being shunned by family members who dislike being brushed aside, these analysands can hold a great fascination for admiring relatives who hope to blow up their own egos in contact with such narcissistic personalities.

Yet analysis shows how little that admiration reassures these analysands; they always need just a tiny bit more, as if, at root, the whole thing was a charade. They sometimes suffer unconsciously from insecurity and a lack of confidence in their own worth, which leads them to keep blowing up their ego even further in a frantic attempt to feel that it is reliable after all. They then have the feeling that they would be better off elsewhere or with other partners, thus giving the impression of ceaselessly wishing to cross and re-cross the same river, as if it were always on the other bank that they would feel better, or as if, by trying even harder, they might at last come to feel that they really existed.

Space without objects gives rise to vertigo

One form of vertigo appears in the following way: patients start suddenly to feel faint when confronting wide open spaces that normally fail to bother them; without any apparent reason this type of space now seems an unbearable void to them. Moreover, it is not merely if it opens up under their feet that this particular void strikes them as being unfathomable, but also if it opens up above them, so much so that one analysand told me: 'I am afraid of falling upwards'. The main characteristic, however, was expressed in this phrase: 'If only something could interrupt my gaze, then my vertigo would go!'

Most frequently though, this type of vertigo appears in the form of dizziness quite unconnected with the perception of an external void, in analysands who had never before been particularly troubled by this condition. Suddenly, these patients feel giddy, and are afraid of having blackouts or losing their balance, conditions for which they usually consult their family physician. Every time this happened to one of my patients, the family doctor, finding no physical cause, simply advised the patient to wait and see; and, in fact, the symptoms always disappeared spontaneously. However, for the analysand no less than for me, the disappearance of these symptoms coincided in a striking manner with the realization of their significance in the analysand's inner history.

Yves: a narcissistic analysand

Several years ago, I was treating a very brilliant patient: Yves seemed to lord it over his family, his friends and his professional associates; everyone seemed to be devoted to him and tried to meet his wishes, as if being in his good books made them more valuable people. In the analysis, without realizing the significance of what he was doing and despite my interventions, he tried to lord it over me as well by arranging the setting of the sessions to his liking, always arriving late and paying me when he pleased; moreover, no matter whether I kept silent or spoke, he always heard me say what he had projected into me and not what I was actually saying. In analysis, as with his family and professional colleagues, he was like Narcissus who, looking at his reflection in a pool, believed that he saw an object distinct from himself, when in fact he was merely gazing at himself.

And yet Yves had asked for analysis because he suffered, in a confused way but all the same profoundly, from not feeling that he was alive. No sign of admiration was great enough to put him at his ease, none managed to convince him of his worth. He loved to go abroad, because he believed that he would feel more himself elsewhere; but he always had to return home quickly since, once he reached his foreign destination, the outside world, where he thought he would feel better, turned as hostile as the place he had left behind. He gave me the impression of 'running after himself' in space, but also in time, because he thought he would be more himself later rather than now.

It was clear to me that the reason why Yves felt unworthy was that he avoided coming up against the limits of others. It was very difficult to put up any resistance to him, because as soon as an object mentioned its own intentions, Yves greeted all such intentions unwittingly with contempt or indifference. I was reminded of Freud's comment (1915c) that when a narcissistic subject discovers the object, he feels hatred for the external world represented by that object. I was quite taken aback by the great fascination Yves exerted on those around him. True, some people got out of his way, but many admired him unconditionally as if, by getting into his good books, they might acquire some of his apparent self-assurance; in any case, most of them seemed to fear that Yves might lose interest in them, as if that were tantamount to being rejected by life itself.

Your home is not my home

There was one very important moment in Yves's psychoanalysis: during one session he said to me: 'I never feel that I am being myself. I never feel at home, not even in my own place, not even here.' By 'not even here', Yves was referring to my consulting room. I replied: 'Perhaps the reason why you cannot feel at home in your own place is that you have failed to realize that here, in my consulting room, you are in my place, not at home. Here in my consulting room, it seems only natural that you should not be feeling at home, because you are not so in fact. Don't you feel that there is a difference between being in the home of others and being in your own place?' Yves then said, sounding surprised: 'I never thought that being here was being in your place.'

I believe that his house and mine were images of our two persons and that he never became aware (even though he knew it rationally) that I was distinct from him, that we had two different homes, and that if he failed to appreciate the difference between being in his place and in mine, he could not possibly appreciate the uniqueness of his own home. Until that time, he had acted as if the boundary between him and the object did not exist, as if the object was an extension of himself; but this absence of a frontier between the ego and the object implied that he did not know clearly where he ended and the other began.

For the next two weeks or so, Yves complained of vertigo. He had the impression that everything around him was swaying. A physician whom he consulted found nothing wrong with him physically. It quickly became clear to Yves that his vertigo was related to what he had discovered during analysis. The realization that I was a separate individual, that I existed outside of him, that I might have needs and wishes differing from his, had caused his view of the world to waver. He then came to appreciate his vulnerability, the loss of his omnipotence, but also to feel that both he and other people existed, even if that existence seemed fragile to him. This transition from his old outlook to his new gave him vertigo. He had reached a moment of radical change; even if the old perspective could not be abandoned at one fell swoop, Yves could not forget what he had caught a glimpse of.

The presence of limits prevents narcissistic haemorrhage

After these two weeks during which Yves reflected on the many aspects of the discoveries he had just made, the vertigo disappeared; Yves turned up for his session, late as usual, and said to me: 'For the first time, I thought of your feelings as I walked through your door. Normally I think: "I'm sure to get told off for being late", even though you have never done that. But this time, I said to myself: "What can she possibly be thinking when she realizes that I haven't turned up yet?"' As he walked through my door, which symbolized the frontier between his person and mine, Yves had come to realize that he did not know my thoughts, that his thoughts were not mine, his feelings not mine, and that therefore he had thoughts and feelings of his own. He realized in particular that those 'tellings off' that he had thought he could hear had not come from me but had been projected into me by him; like Echo, the nymph who fell in love with Narcissus, he had been hearing the echo of his own voice, which had stopped him from hearing mine. Now he tried to hear what I was actually saying. My thoughts, as distinct from his, began to interest him; he could start toing and froing between what was his and what was mine, so that an exchange of views became possible. A few days later, when he handed me my fee for the past month, he said: 'I am still paying you late, but for the first time I thought that you might need the money.' I replied: 'I have the feeling that I am becoming a person in your eyes, and that you have begun to realize that you might be a person for me.' In effect, I had the impression that before Yves could accept that he was coming up against my separate identity, he had to feel there was something in it for him, that something being the feeling that he was a person, that he had a life of his own.

In the past, Yves had tried to ignore the boundary between the ego and the object, a boundary symbolized in space by my door and in time by the beginning of the session: he had actually looked upon it as a gap between us and not as a link facilitating communication between our two beings; but above all he had considered that boundary as a restraint placed on him. Now he had discovered that the boundary could allow him to know his shape and hence to define himself. 'The boundaries of the ego and those of the object had been experienced as putting an end to the narcissistic haemorrhage and not as the rejection of one person by another, or, what is worse, as indifference' (D. Quinodoz 1989b: 1650).

Diane: 'I can't stop thinking'

When Diane started her analysis, she showed signs of tireless activity culminating in dizziness. She had chosen a very absorbing profession in which she devoted herself to others unstintingly. One aspect of her request for analysis involved this complaint: 'I simply cannot stop . . .'. The complaint had become even more acute when, instead of associating it with action, Diane placed it on the psychic level: 'I cannot stop *thinking*'. I said to myself that she was twisting and turning like a screw, but, despite her turbulent ways, she found the time to keep arriving punctually for her four weekly sessions. In analysis, Diane proved to be a very interesting person, warm and vivacious, but at the beginning of the analysis she often introduced the rhythm which I imagined went with her professional activity: her free associations were gradually transformed into an increasingly rapid succession of ideas, so much so that her speech accelerated, rose and filled the room, leaving me not the least chink for intervention. My attempts to get a word in edgeways were either brushed aside or went unnoticed. I then gained the impression that Diane's ego had become hypertrophied by exponential expansion that she could no longer control, and that threatened to swallow every object in its path.

It seemed perfectly clear to me that Diane's swollen discourse during analytical sessions was an instance of narcissistic haemorrhage. It was as if Diane's ego became hypertrophied at the same time as her speech; but the louder her voice, the more diluted became her ego, which thus lost its organizing power, that is its essence. Diane doubtless thought she was speaking to *me*, but her speech was not addressed to me as a person but disseminated into an objectless world. I understood why she complained of being unable to stop thinking: her spillage of thoughts into an unresisting world robbed her of the pleasure of thinking in more stimulating ways. Clearly, during those sessions, Diane did not feel that there was the least boundary between her and me, no dividing line facilitating a dialogue. Besides, she sometimes walked into my place without ringing the bell and her dearest wish was to be able to proceed straight into my consulting room through the walls of the building, without crossing the boundaries put up by the front door, the passage and the waiting room. In that way, she hoped not to come up against the limits of the object, although she realized that without the resistance of the object she was in danger of losing her self.

This attitude during analysis seemed a repetition of what Diane complained she experienced in her profession. But how could I possibly have described as narcissistic the activities of a woman who ceaselessly devoted herself to others? It was because that overbrimming activity, self-fuelled by growing excitation, struck me as taking little account of others as personalized, independent objects. Were the others perhaps a mere pretext justifying the ever-expanding activity Diane needed in order to gain the feeling that she existed? To me they appeared as the projection of the fragile personality Diane was at that moment, and of which she took care through others. She was like Narcissus, who gazed tenderly at his reflection in the water without realizing that he was looking at himself.

An object able to halt thought

During these 'haemorrhagic' sessions, I tried not to be carried away by this whirlpool; I tried to remain centred in myself and to feel calm in order to remain an object available for Diane. However, during one of the sessions, I was surprised to discover quite suddenly that my thoughts kept straying from what was happening in the session. I asked myself why this might be. I had already had the same feeling of escaping in thought from Luc, but my counter-transference had been quite different with him. I tried to discover what was behind it all: if Diane had arranged things unconsciously so as to draw me into her whirlpool during the session to the point that I was afraid of disappearing, had she perhaps done so in order to make me understand her problems? Might my fear of disappearing, which I had experienced thanks to her unconscious attitude towards me during the session, not be a reflection of her own fear?

It was then that I deliberately interrupted Diane's swirling discourse by saying: 'I keep looking for you; you tell me a great many things, but I have the feeling that I'll never be able find you yourself amidst all these interesting topics.'

My intervention had several aims; I wanted first of all to stake out my boundaries and to do that in such a way that Diane's thought came up against mine; but I also did not want to leave it at differentiating myself from Diane by refusing to become a whirlpool like her. In order to take my boundaries into consideration she would have to realize that doing so was in her own interest and in particular that I did not resist her in order to lose her but in order to find her. By saying 'I am looking for you', I was hoping to make her feel that I was not just looking after myself, but also trying to find her. Moreover, by telling her about my feeling of losing her in her torrent of words I tried to indicate that her mental agitation might not be an essential facet of her personality and that she might perhaps try to differentiate her real personality from the whirlpool. But that was something Diane alone was able to do.

She suddenly calmed down and told me that all this reminded her that her mother had come to see her the night before, and that she had realized that she could not bear her mother because she 'twisted and turned like a screw'. She sensed that as soon as she was in her mother's presence she stopped being able to think, her ideas being blown away like so much fluff by her mother's agitation. Her mother, on the other hand, seemed never to be lost for thought, talking in 'operational' terms. She added that in contact with her mother she herself, without realizing it, had been forced to 'spin like a top', something she also had the impression of doing in her professional life. She added that she could not see herself stopping this sort of behaviour, because 'when a top stops spinning it falls down'.

She was all the more surprised to notice that during this session she had managed to stop the top. That showed her that the top, the screw, was her way of picturing her mother, that the top was not really herself, and that moreover she now knew that the reason why she was so keen on her analytic sessions was that she sometimes discovered a rhythm in analysis that helped her to stop the top, and hence to feel that she was being herself. During this session, Diane had thus had the intense experience of differentiating herself from the analyst-object, and from the mother-object.

Vertigo

Next day Diane telephoned me because she felt unable to leave her bed and to come for her session; the whole room was spinning round her, and she was having a dreadful bout of vertigo. Her doctor had found nothing wrong with her physically. Two days later, the giddiness having abated, Diane was able to come for her session. She said that she had thought hard about our last session and had mulled it over a lot, because she had become convinced that there was a link between that last session and her giddiness. She said: 'I realized to what large extent I had confused myself with my mother; it was she who was the screw or the top, not I. Now I have the feeling that I have got rid of the screw and the top, I no longer turn like a screw, but for two whole days I felt that the outside world was spinning round me.' It was as if Diane had created a boundary separating her mother from herself.

Three days later the giddiness had completely disappeared. A little while later still, Diane had changed direction even in her profession, opting for an activity that involved a calmer rhythm and one, moreover, in which she felt that she could relate to others. In Yves's language, we might say that Diane had place a door between her house and her mother's.

Expansion-related vertigo appears during the sudden transition from an unlimited representation of the inner world to a limited representation

I would like to stress first of all that it is for the sake of a clearer exposition that I speak schematically of a world without limits, or without an object, and of a world with limits or filled with objects. Clearly, I am referring to tendencies, to asymptotic processes, because no one can live in a world in which there is no object or no limit. In particular, the analysands I have been discussing were far too advanced to think otherwise.

I have chosen the cases of Diane and Yves, who seemed to me especially representative, but I could equally well have mentioned several other narcissistic analysands who felt giddy the moment they became aware that their inner malaise was connected with the expansion of their ego in a world without an object, and began to sense that by putting a frontier between the objects and themselves they could stop the narcissistic haemorrhage. This new view of their internal world entailed so great a transformation that, while establishing a new internal equilibrium, they were forced to project the feeling that their internal world wobbled to the outside. It is worth noting that for Diane the internal world was in double turmoil because in a sense she had become used to the picture of a turbulent internal world that she had taken over from her mother, and because she was getting rid of it to find a calmer internal world of her own.

The appearance of vertigo during the transition from a world without limits to a world *with* limits has at least two explanations. *On the one hand*, the awareness that there are limits between ego and objects entails a new representation of the internal world, which is in stark contrast to the earlier, anxiety-ridden representation of an unlimited world in which nothing could stop the ego's expansion. Before arriving at that realization, the analysand, accustomed to his representation of an unlimited internal world, merely felt faint or dizzy without knowing why. *On the other hand*, the renunciation of an unlimited world in favour of a limited world introduces a measure of anxiety, because every choice means taking a risk and losing a known advantage for untested benefits.

It is only natural then that the analysand should wonder whether the advantages of a *limited* world will provide enough compensation for his renunciation of the familiar advantages of the *unlimited* world. On this subject, without entering more fully into Diane's and Yves's analyses, I have precisely referred to the fact, that in both cases, the narcissistic haemorrhage had at least the provisional advantage of making it possible for both patients to hide, as if under a thick fog, a frightening facet of their lives which, unconsciously, they hoped to exclude from their personal history. Entering a limited world meant fitting that facet into their limited internal world and to remember it.

André Green dealt with this problem in his *Narcissisme de vie, narcissisme de mort*, and has proposed the following solution:

> The problem is to realize just how much the advantages introduced by the limit can offset the disadvantages of losing the unlimited by separating

what is now one side from the other. That is, by constructing something other, a difference. The solution is on the one hand to ensure the consistency of the two territories, and on the other hand to find a way of allowing them to communicate without becoming trapped in the dilemma of invasion and evasion, that is of the loss of the neighbourhood, the loss of the neighbour – the Other.

(1983: 163)

8

Competition-related vertigo

Anxiety about surpassing the oedipal rival

Competition-related vertigo can assume different forms but always remains the equivalent of anxiety related to oedipal rivalry, and in particular to the phantasy of surpassing one's rival; it is, for instance, the vertigo associated with climbing up a ladder, of being 'too' high while imagining others well below one, of overtaking people in a car or in some other way, or, in certain cases, of watching another person approach the void. In the last case, in fact, the person who has vertigo imagines that the other is about to fall: he is dropping him in his imagination.

An oedipal context: the presence of two distinct parents

When Luc told me that there was a sea between the islands and that he could swim (which meant that between sessions there was a relational space he could use to communicate), he was voicing a complex feeling, all of whose implications he did not grasp at once. But Luc came to realize gradually, by means of word play, that the dynamic relational space he called the sea (*la mer*) was also a symbolic expression of the permanence of the mother (*la mère*): the mother who, in the transference, had become a continuous object for Luc, and this despite the discontinuity of the analytic sessions, an object that retained its essential characteristics and importance even during long absences. Luc no longer needed the concrete presence of the mother to realize that she was precious to him; precious, that is, because the role she played in his life, be it agreeable or not, was an important one. As a result, he also came to appreciate that his own role was an important part in his mother's life.

At the same time, the father appeared: Luc discovered that the father had

84

been present from the very start, be it only in the mother's phantasies, in the psychic space that symbolically represented the permanence of the *mother*. In Chapter 6, when discussing the appearance of internal space, we have already outlined the emergence of the father: the patient imagines him as either carrying a limp child (easily dropped) or a tonic child (easier to carry).

In fact, inasmuch as their representations of psychic space are very blurred, these analysands refer mainly to a fairly undifferentiated mother; it would be more correct to say that they refer to a maternal object in which mother and father are confused, a single blurred object of indistinct sex (a father-mother). One of my patients always spoke of her 'daddy-mummy' as if her parents were a single person. That representation which glosses over the incompleteness of the mother, deprives her of her desires and of the power of her drives: if she is complete, she has nothing left to desire.

By contrast, when the image of a mother playing her specific role, and her specific sexual role in particular, appears, everything changes: the mother does not have everything; she is seen as someone distinct from the father; she has only one sex; she needs the father to have children; in short, she is no longer omnipotent and can desire the father. What she loses in illusory omnipotence, she gains in existential power, limited but real, and especially in the dynamism of her drives and in the richness of her desires. It is no longer her idealized image that is being appreciated but *simply* this particular mother, this mother *as she really is*. The child discovers that his mother cannot be *this mother* without being *this* woman, that is, without conjuring up the presence of the father. As a result, better communication can be established between the analysand and his internal mother, since, in losing her illusory, idealized character the mother is henceforth considered to be *simply herself*, thus leaving the child with the possibility of being *simply itself*.

The symbolic meaning of competition-related vertigo

The father's presence thus emerges quite naturally during these moments of analysis, and it is then that a new form of vertigo can be discerned. It reflects an oedipal problem: with the arrival of a third party, competition has become possible. Feelings of oedipal guilt appear, and the oedipal conflict may usher in competition-related vertigo. It is no longer a type of vertigo reflecting anxiety about losing one's own identity, or about being dropped or absorbed by the object, but vertigo expressing castration anxiety. In fact, in this context, the wish to 'drop' the beloved third party in order to take his place or to conquer him makes the patient phantasize that the father is plotting revenge; might not his wish to drop the father (or his substitute) entail his own fall by an act of retaliation? Vertigo may then emerge as an alarm signal warning the patient against fulfilling desires whose consequences strike him as being dangerous: the patient's vertigo stops him from even thinking that he could climb higher up the ladder than his father.

Competition-related vertigo does not cut into the integrity of the ego

With competition-related vertigo, we enter the register of neurotic defence mechanisms. In some cases, this form of vertigo may coexist with other forms that we have already discussed and hence bear witness to the presence of different levels of integration in one and the same person. If, on the other hand, competition-related vertigo appears as a new form of vertigo in a patient who used to present other forms of vertigo, we would be right to think that a regressive part of that patient may have developed in such a way that he no longer has any need for that particular split, and that he now adopts, in a more extensive manner, secondary neurotic defence mechanisms in better tune with external reality.

Competition-related vertigo may sometimes prove a real nuisance to the patient, for example if the symptoms are very acute, if they are triggered off very easily, or again if the patient meets the conditions bringing out this type of vertigo in his daily life; however, this type of vertigo is never as troublesome as the others because it does not undermine the patient's sense of being himself or of existing in his own right, as happens, for example, with vertigo related to annihilation anxiety.

Competition-related vertigo appears in analysands who believe that they are distinct from the object; they feel that the existence of differences between them and the object is a precondition of the personalization of their own and the object's existence, and of possible exchanges between the two. Such analysands, distinct from the object, no longer have a vital need for a containing object or external carrier because they have internalized it in their psychic space. They have discovered, by introjective identification with their mother or father, or in their transference on to the analyst, their own active capacity to contain themselves. Here I distinguish introjective from narcissistic identification: narcissistic identification involves a confusion of identities and threatens to rob the subject of his personality through his unconscious desire to be the object; it confuses subject and object in causing the disappearance of the specificity of one or the other, or of both at once. Introjective identification, on the other hand, leaves the object completely intact while allowing the subject to be himself more and more; in that case the presence of the object is a revealing factor enabling the subject to become aware of his own capacity to be in contact with those of the object.

86

Conditions for the emergence of competition-related vertigo

These conditions involve the love and hate relations between the analysand and the object. This type of vertigo appears when 'the ego begins to distinguish love from hatred of the same object, but cannot be sure of being able to connect them' (D. Quinodoz 1987: 1591). That moment, even if unaccompanied by competition-related vertigo, has always struck me as being very important in therapy; I believe that it corresponds to the appearance, in Kleinian theory, of the depressive position before its elaboration, and, in Freudian theory, to the moment when the analysand, though already capable of presenting genital ambivalence, has not yet resolved his Oedipus complex. But what do we mean by distinguishing love from hatred and by connecting these affects?

Different meanings of the word 'love'

According to Freud, *love opposed to indifference* must be distinguished from *love opposed to hate*. *Love* opposed to indifference is itself made up of *love* and hate. In fact, 'loving and hating taken together are the opposite of the condition of unconcern or indifference' (1915c: 133), which Freud contrasts with (total) love. Freud thus attaches two meanings to the word 'love': on the one hand, total love, opposed to indifference and made up of love and hate; and on the other hand, a love that is a component of total love and is the opposite of hate.

Love opposed to indifference

Freud states that, at the beginning of life, there is neither love nor hate of the object – there is *indifference*.

> At this time the external world is not cathected with interest (in a general sense) and is indifferent for purposes of satisfaction. During this period, therefore, the ego-subject coincides with what is pleasurable and the external world with what is indifferent (or possibly unpleasurable, as being a source of stimulation). If for the moment we define loving as the relation of the ego to its sources of pleasure, the situation in which the ego loves itself only and is indifferent to the external world illustrates the first of the opposites which we found to 'loving'.
>
> (Freud 1915c: 135)

This indifference to the object, or failure to invest the object with interest, corresponds to Freud's description of the oceanic feeling (1930a) due to which the infant, in its confusion with the non–ego, does not know where its ego stops and the non–ego begins; Freud then goes on to show how the ego emerges from the non–ego by discovering hatred for what is not the ego, in such a way that the love–hate directed at the object becomes differentiated from indifference to it.

The difference between Freud's uncathected object and Melanie Klein's indistinct pre-natal object does not strike me as being very great; to my mind, there is a much greater difference in their attitude to the ego, which is more active with Melanie Klein; for her, the ego projects and introjects, and differentiates itself actively from the object; it enacts the duality of the drives which it detects through the affects of love and hate.

Love opposed to hate

'When, during the stage of primary narcissism, the object makes its appearance, the second opposite of loving, namely hating, also attains its development' (Freud 1915c: 136). This, to Freud, is the 'object stage' where 'pleasure and unpleasure signify relations of the ego to the object' (*ibid*.: 137). When the object becomes a source of pleasure we say that we *love* it. Conversely, when the object is the source of unpleasure we *hate* it.

Freud uses the term '*purified pleasure ego*' to refer to a new development of the ego under the domination of the pleasure principle: 'In so far as the objects which are presented to it are sources of pleasure, it [the ego] takes them into itself, "introjects" them (to use Ferenczi's term) and, on the other hand, it expels whatever within itself becomes a source of unpleasure' (*ibid*.: 136). It seems to me that, albeit from a different perspective, Freud is here describing a psychic mechanism close to the splitting processes Melanie Klein associates with the paranoid-schizoid position.

The love–hate confusion

For Freud, the opposition between love and hate is not established all at once, and is not really reached before the genital stage. As long as the object is only desired to satisfy partial drives, we cannot say whether the ego loves or hates it, so closely fused are love and hate; in that case the effect on the object is more or less the same, regardless of whether it is due to love or hate: in fact, oral love devours, anal love imprisons or expels, and the object may be mainly interested in not being devoured or imprisoned, and cares little whether that be through love or hatred. Those who devour or imprison the object 'out of love' do not bother about the effect their love has on an object; they thus treat it as a part object. I think that it is in this sense that

Freud writes: 'the attitudes of love and hate cannot be made use of for the relations of instincts to their objects, but are reserved for the relations of the total ego to objects' (*ibid.*: 137); we cannot say that the ego feels love for milk or the breast (an object desired to satisfy the partial drive); by contrast we can say that it feels love or hate for the food-providing mother (a total person). From this I infer that total love, as opposed to indifference, and itself composed of love and hate, can assume very different forms depending on the relationship between the love and the hate elements composing it.

Two forms of ambivalence

This inference led me to distinguish two forms of ambivalence, which I have called pregenital and genital ambivalence respectively (D. Quinodoz 1987). It seemed to me that Freud took this distinction into account implicitly, even though he failed to conceptualize it explicitly. In effect, Freud mentions cases in which the affects of love and hate cannot be distinguished because they are too closely blended. For me, what we have here is a *pregenital form of ambivalence*: 'Love in this form and at this preliminary stage is hardly to be distinguished from hate in its attitude towards the object' (Freud 1915c: 139). A child, for instance, can feel devouring or imprisoning love for its mother; if it is of an age when that kind of love prevails, the mother will, in general, allow herself to be 'devoured' or 'imprisoned' by a baby who makes demands on her time and energy; but when the child has grown older, she will no longer allow it to treat her as a part object that satisfies oral or anal partial drives.

Occasionally, though, Freud speaks of a quite different form of ambivalence, which I have called *genital ambivalence*, for instance when he describes the feelings of 'Little Hans'. Here he uses *ambivalent love* to refer to a 'well-grounded love and a no less justifiable hatred directed towards one and the same person' (Freud 1926d: 102). Freud was referring to the genital love of someone who had resolved or was about to resolve the conflict resulting from oedipal ambivalence by acknowledging clearly differentiated feelings of love and hatred towards the same object; these affects, love and hate, can then be *linked* because they have been *distinguished* from each other. 'Not until the genital organization is established does love become the opposite of hate' (Freud 1915c: 139).

These two forms of ambivalent love are quite different: in pregenital ambivalence 'loving and hating cannot be associated because they are confused'; in genital ambivalence, 'love and hate are linked because they are distinct, which facilitates love of the total object by the total ego' (D. Quinodoz 1987: 1591). In this *association*, each element preserves its specificity, while being linked to the other to constitute a whole larger than each constituent element; when they are *mixed up* each element loses its specificity and disappears in the whole. Here we are back with a general principle: we must be able to distinguish before we can combine. Without a prior distinction, we end up with confusion, not combination. It is when the son feels ambivalent genital love for his father that he can go on to distinguish between what he likes and what he detests about this important figure. Ambivalent genital love strikes me as being a concept close to the Kleinian view of the elaboration of the depressive position, when the total person represents much more for the subject than any of the facets added together.

A third form of ambivalence: transitional ambivalence; competition-related vertigo appears when there is a juxtaposition of love and hate (but neither confusion nor association of these affects)

The position of the son who feels 'a well-founded love and a no less justifiable hatred' towards his father does not necessarily imply a synthesis of these affects. I believe that there is an intermediate position, namely the juxtaposition of the affects: the son may be capable of distinguishing love from hatred instead of confusing them, but still not know what to do with that distinction; before realizing that he can link his love and hatred for his father, he can pass through a very anxious stage of transitional ambivalent love in which the terms of the ambivalence are juxtaposed. Now, in my view, it is at this critical moment that competition-related vertigo may appear.

I feel it is important to stress how much the approach of Freud and Klein, who differ in some theoretical respects, can converge at the level of clinical interpretation. In fact, I find that, in both cases, there is a crucial factor corresponding, in Melanie Klein, to the not-yet-elaborated depressive position and, in Freud, to pregenital ambivalence before the resolution of the Oedipus complex. In both cases, the patient is filled with anxiety when he becomes aware of the duality of the drives and can see no way of linking them up.

A clinical example of competition-related vertigo

In the course of his analysis, Luc came gradually to realize that 'the' vertigo from which he suffered could assume different forms, which he was able to distinguish because they carried distinct meanings; after several years of analysis, some of these forms, namely the most regressive and the most unbearable, had disappeared, but competition-related vertigo now came to the fore in its specific form. In fact, Luc had never been able to climb a ladder; the mere idea of doing so gave him vertigo, though it was only now that he began to grasp the reason why. His father had used a ladder in his professional work. Luc remembered that, as a child, he had phantasized kicking his father's ladder away, and he now relived the associated anxiety: how could he possibly want the father he so admired to fall off? During analysis, he started to imagine that he was at the wheel of his immense car, overtaking me as I was trundling along in my little one; then the scene changed: he was on top of the ladder while I, his father, remained below. What might I do in these circumstances? Kick the ladder to make him fall off? It now became clear to Luc that this last phantasy expressed his fear that the analyst, his father in the transference, might castrate him to stop him from surpassing him. This phantasy helped him to take stock of the oedipal rivalry and castration anxiety present in the transference.

His phantasy echoing back to an oedipal problem and to castration anxiety was moreover connected with other pre-oedipal phantasies that suddenly began to make sense at several levels at once. In fact, Luc discovered that his occasional nostalgic wish to return to his mother's womb, which seemed a purely pre-oedipal desire, not only recalled his refusal to be born, but also the refusal to be born 'little'. In other words, side by side with more regressive wishes, he also had the wish to have been born the biggest of all, and bigger than his father in particular. Luc realized that he had been unconsciously afraid of being found out wishing to usurp his father's place. That stopped him from enjoying his successes, because they invariably seemed so many phantasized realizations of his desire to steal successes that were not his due. His anxiety when overtaking other cars was a fear of rivalry. It was then that he began to sense that competition-related vertigo might well have served him as a provisional means of unconsciously avoiding being caught in the act of stealing his father's place and being punished for it: he was in no danger of rising above his father because his vertigo stopped him.

Not long after this realization, Luc burst out laughing at the start of a session: that very morning he had been able to climb a big ladder. At first, he had, as usual, stayed at the bottom, allowing his colleagues to go up first. But then a latecomer came running up and said with obvious relief: 'How very kind of you to wait for me, I would never have known which way to go!', and then Luc had no trouble in climbing the ladder himself. It was as if, prepared by the discovery he had made not so long before, the act of climbing the ladder had quite suddenly ceased to be a symbol of oedipal rivalry. Since this new meaning did not entail a castration threat, Luc no longer had to guard against it – he could dispense with the vertigo alarm signal. The symbol had recovered its momentum: climbing as high as or higher than his father could have other meanings than dethroning him.

This clinical example confirmed my belief that competition-related vertigo does not reflect anxiety about the destruction of the ego or about the loss of a vital object, but is a sign of anxiety about losing the love of the object or the love of the super-ego entailing castration anxiety.

Competition-related vertigo from a feminine perspective

Can women have competition-related vertigo?

I have used the case of a male patient to illustrate competition-related vertigo; I added that this type of vertigo must be placed at the oedipal level and was most often a manifestation of castration anxiety. Now, Freud said in 'Anxiety and Instinctual Life':

> Fear of castration is not, of course, the only motive for repression: indeed, it finds no place in women, for though they have a castration complex they cannot have a fear of being castrated. Its place is taken in their sex by a fear of loss of love, which is evidently a later prolongation of the infant's anxiety if it finds its mother absent.
>
> (1933a: 87)

Does that mean that women cannot have competition-related vertigo, seeing that, according to Freud, they have no fear of being castrated?

I must admit that competition-related vertigo did not seem to manifest itself in my male and female analysands in identical fashion; it was mainly the men who presented competition-related vertigo; the women complained of it less often, which does not mean that they did not suffer from it. I have met female analysands who mentioned in the course of their analysis that they had vertigo when climbing a ladder, or when seeing one of their close relatives leaning over a balcony; this was usually brought up as a trivial subsidiary symptom and never as a reason for analysis. While no generalization can be based on that observation, I must mention that I was struck by the different attitude of male and female patients to this form of vertigo. Thus, during a trip to Mexico I noticed that some people in our group, men and women, never climbed the pyramids; these persons had vertigo; but while the men expressed their disappointment at not being able to climb up, most of the women who had vertigo simply said that they did not feel like climbing and talked calmly below while watching the others go up. I found this observation interesting, even though it might very well have been the result of a combination of very particular circumstances.

For the rest, it is clear to me that female analysands can have competition-related vertigo situated at the oedipal level just like male patients. However, since women do not have a penis, they cannot fear that it will be cut off, and their anxiety about their drives could not possibly be fuelled by that threat. Are these two claims incompatible?

Penis envy

Freud attributes a castration complex to little girls no less than to little boys, but stresses that its content is different. According to Freud, the little boy experiences the castration complex as a consequence of *castration anxiety*, while the little girl experiences it as a consequence of *penis envy*. 'Girls hold their mother responsible for their lack of penis and do not forgive her for their being thus put at a disadvantage' (Freud 1933*a*: 124). The girl sometimes thinks the penis she desires might still grow or that she could obtain one, and

> continues to hold on for a long time to the wish to get something like it herself and she believes in that possibility for improbably long years; and analysis can show that, at a period when knowledge of reality has long since rejected the fulfilment of the wish as unattainable, it persists in the unconscious and retains a considerable cathexis of energy.
>
> (*ibid.*: 125)

Analysis also shows that, in some cases, the chase after success or the pursuit of an intellectual profession may well appear in some women as 'a sublimated modification of this repressed wish' (*ibid.*: 168).

Freud's view of the castration complex and of the Oedipus complex in girls

For Freud, awareness of the lack of a penis leads girls to feel that they are less worthy than boys, and they extend this depreciation to women in general and to their mothers in particular. Girls accordingly repudiate their love for their mother, thus paving the way for oedipal hostility towards her. In effect, disappointed at not having received a penis from her mother, the girl turns to her father expecting him to give her a baby, which represents a penis equivalent for her. 'With the transference of the wish for a penis-baby on to her father, the girl has entered the situation of the Oedipus complex' (*ibid.*: 129). In the event, the mother becomes a rival who obtains from the father the penis-baby he refuses his daughter.

Freud goes on to show that, when it comes to the Oedipus complex, there is some difference between the sexes.

93

[In girls] the castration complex prepares for the Oedipus complex instead of destroying it; the girl is driven out of her attachment to her mother through the influence of envy for the penis and she enters the Oedipus situation as though into a haven of refuge. In the absence of fear of castration the chief motive is lacking which leads boys to surmount the Oedipus complex. Girls remain in it for an indeterminate length of time; they demolish it late and, even so, incompletely.

(*ibid.*: 129)

Freud contends that the man who turns from his mother to his wife is relieved of his fear of castration, while the woman who turns from her father to her husband is not relieved of her penis envy: she continues to demand from her husband the penis-baby she once claimed from her father: the man's fear of castration has disappeared, but not the woman's penis envy.

I consider this Freudian analysis of penis envy, which can be verified in therapy, very important, but only on one condition: that its partial aspect is borne in mind. When Freud concluded that women, unlike men, never completely abandon their Oedipus complex, he may well have suspected that one of the reasons for it might have been that his argument failed to take all aspects of female sexuality into account. Various psychoanalysts, especially Melanie Klein, Janine Chasseguet-Smirgel (1964), Joyce McDougall (1964) and many others have made complementary contributions to the understanding of female sexuality which must not be overlooked. I do not wish to discuss post-Freudian contributions to this field in any great detail; in what follows I shall simply present my own point of view inasmuch as it may throw light on competition-related vertigo in the specific form it takes in women.

An equivalent of castration anxiety in small girls

When I characterized competition-related vertigo as a manifestation of castration anxiety, I attributed it to women as well as to men: actually, I believe that, in small girls, there is no castration anxiety in the strict sense, that is, no fear of having the male sex organ cut off, but there is an equivalent anxiety, namely the fear of having the female sex organ amputated.

I am not the first to think that Freud's analysis of the castration complex in girls seems to bear on just one aspect of female sexuality. Freud might give the impression that one of the chief characteristics of the female sex is the absence of a penis; this would suggest that one considers women as men deprived of their penis, and hence as persons without a sex organ, that is, with nothing. In that case, women would be persons not only deprived of male genitals, but of female genitals as well. Now, women can admittedly

94

have penis envy, much as men can have envy of the female genitals, as manifested, for instance, in envy of child-bearing; but they can also be afraid of having their own (female) genitals amputated, much as men can be afraid of castration.

If we ignore their fear of having their genitals amputated, we place women in a doubly delicate situation: not only, like every human being, must they accept that they lack the genitals of the opposite sex, but they must also behave as if they were not afraid of having the organs they do own amputated, because the existence of these organs is passed over in silence or might even be considered the result of a negative hallucination. Passing in silence over the fact that a woman might be afraid of having her own genitals amputated might give the impression that the very existence of the feminine genitals is being doubted, and that strikes me as an amputation threat in itself, not unlike the castration threat in men. The fact that the female genitals are invisible, or hardly visible, is not enough to justify the view that they are not recognized intuitively by the little girl, because there is such a thing as proprioceptive perception of invisible organs, and also phantasy knowledge of one's own body image underpinned by the mother's reverie and the attitude of the child's family. Moreover, Freud mentions 'premonitory sensations' concerning the existence of the vagina and of sexual intercourse when discussing the case of Little Hans (1909b: 134).

In the analysis of some of my women patients I realized how much the negative hallucination of the female genitals had affected those women who had the impression that the sexuality of a human being can only be defined positively by the presence of a penis, the opposite sex being characterized by its absence. The moment they discover in analysis, with great relief, that they are human beings without a penis *but* with female genitals, they realize that their lack of a penis gives them the advantage of having female genitals together with the wish to receive (not to possess) the partner's penis; could then at long last discover how unjustifiably low an opinion they had had of themselves, having equated their lack of a penis with being 'holed', *being empty, a mere nothing.*

One of the consequences of this disparaging attitude was double hostility towards their mother, disparaged in her turn for having failed to give them either male or female genitals; but above all the tendency to consider their own children, actual or potential, as penis-babies, substitutes for their own lack of virility and narcissistic-phantasy extensions of themselves, instead of considering them as independent persons, each having their own life. The moment these children, who serve their mother as a penis, leave her to live their own lives, there is high drama: a part of the mother has been cut off and she is left without a penis. Now, the departure of children from home produces quite a different reaction if these children have been treated as separate, whole persons: since their mother does not need them to feel that she is in one piece, they can leave without making her fear that part of herself has been amputated; this in no way detracts from the pain of the separation, but decreases the mother's anxiety at having been left incomplete, and the child's guilt.

The little girl's fear of being amputated by the oedipal rival

If then we take the little girl's own genitals into consideration, the oedipal context assumes a different form from that suggested by Freud; the female situation gets closer to the situation Freud observed in boys. When competing with their mother for the father's love, little girls do indeed fear retaliatory amputation, but amputation of their female genitals and not of a penis. This threat to their femininity can take various, more or less psychic and more or less somatic, forms: the feeling of being unattractive, the inability to give birth to children biologically or symbolically, the compulsion to repeat an oedipal scene in which they constantly abandon the partner to the rival, or on the contrary are only interested in stealing him from her, the inhibition of their orgasm, psychic sterility or infertility, the feeling of being empty and unable to contain any riches. This last feeling can go hand in hand with corporeal sensations: many women trying to describe their vertigo say that they feel as if their innards were being ripped out of them. This retaliation threat, that is, the amputation of the female genitals of which they had wanted to strip their mothers unconsciously, seems to be of the same order as male castration anxiety.

The fear of having the female genitals amputated combined with penis envy

This female equivalent of castration anxiety becomes more complicated if it is combined with persistent penis envy. In that case, the rival whom the (female) patient is afraid of surpassing is the one who has a penis. The analysand fears, unconsciously, that her success would be ascribed by her family to her being endowed with a penis substitute; she is afraid that this might be considered a deception and that she might be mocked by her family with: 'She is trying to fool us into thinking that she has a penis!' In that case, the lack of a penis may even be felt to be a preventive form of punishment. These patients believe that they have been doubly amputated: not only have they been deprived of the coveted penis, but they also have the feeling that they lack female genitals. The are doubly 'without anything'.

In the course of an analysis we can often observe how male and female patients extend their psychic knowledge of female and male sexuality (the two going hand in hand): at first they may imagine the female body as being 'holed', the female genitals being referred to as a hole (a mere nothing, through which the female empties herself and which prevents her from retaining anything), reflecting the absence of a penis and of any other organ; then they start to imagine the female genitals as a cavity, that is, an active hollow organ that can retain and expel; this organ has a complex relationship with the person as a whole, participates in complex object relationships and makes it possible for its owner to engage in creative activity. This development of the representations of the female genitals goes hand in hand with a development of the representations of the male genitals, because it is quite obvious that virile penetration does not have an object-relational significance if it is achieved in a hole.

Competition-related vertigo in women

Finally, women presenting oedipal competition-related vertigo seem to me to feel less strongly and clearly than men that they have climbed too high, higher than their (male or female) rival, and hence that they are in danger of falling off. Instead they tend to have the unpleasant vertiginous sensation that a hole or a hollow is opening up and imploding inside them, nailing them down. I believe that this reflects a corporeal basis comparable to the primary sensation in men that the amputation of their genitals leaves them empty. Every manifestation of competition-related vertigo in female analysands can have two meanings, depending on whether they are more afraid of having their female genitals amputated or more subject to penis envy. I shall be demonstrating this double meaning in greater detail by giving examples of various forms of competition-related vertigo in female analysands.

Competition-related vertigo and inhibition of curiosity

The giddy feeling that a hollow is opening up inside her and nailing her down can often restrain a woman from the wish to explore or to discover things, as if the aggression that goes with curiosity might elicit retaliation. The inhibition of curiosity is often justified with numerous rationalizations, for instance insistence on the danger a woman runs when studying or travelling far away from her mother, or the belief that fieldwork would stop her from having a husband and children. It is often the hidden aspect of the female genitals that links competition-related vertigo in women to the inhibition of curiosity. In some cases, exploring the world, for instance psychically by engaging in certain studies or professional activities, or physically by travelling far afield, may give rise to vertigo and hence immobilize the patient in advance. In fact, what the young girl attacks in her phantasies about her mother are her hidden genitals, and what she believes is threatened in herself is deeply hidden inside as well. This doubtless gives rise to the feeling that the mere fact of trying to grasp what is hidden constitutes an attempt at amputation, is therefore reprehensible and invites amputation by way of retaliation.

However, in some female patients, this inhibition of curiosity may go hand in hand with penis envy and with the anxiety that one's family circle (parent substitutes) might find out that, for these patients, displaying a curious and adventurous spirit is a way of parading a penis equivalent.

Competition-related vertigo and the inhibition of the wish to make progress

The vertigo linked to the feeling of climbing *higher*, concretely on a ladder or symbolically on the social scale, may also be associated with the fear of having one's female genitals amputated by the mother and being left empty, as if *climbing* were tantamount to boasting about the value of one's own genitals to one's mother and exposing them to her – the rival's – jealous regard. Vertigo, sometimes in the form of 'stage fright', often seems to stop an analysand from showing publicly what her feminine creative capacity can achieve; she stays at the bottom of the ladder, safe from her mother's rival looks, which she believes are envious and destructive.

This inhibition can also occur, albeit with a different significance, in patients presenting penis envy. Through their vertigo they betray the fear that their envy might be discovered if they were caught climbing higher than their rival endowed with a penis, the father or his substitute; this rival may sometimes be the mother as well, phantasized as a phallic woman.

Vertigo and wealth

Vertigo associated with the display of one's wealth is also a form of competition-related vertigo, one by which the female analysand can defend herself from the danger of competing with her mother. I have previously described the toing and froing between transference and counter-transference with a female analysand who presented herself as being poor, without resources, so poverty-stricken in fact that I was tempted to ask her for such modest fees that, had I succumbed to this temptation, I should have colluded with her by encouraging her to rob me. But then the meaning of her alleged poverty dawned on me: she 'unconsciously adopted the air of a poor girl lest I thought of robbing her of riches she clearly did not possess' (D. Quinodoz 1984b: 746). In fact, her outer show of poverty was the expression of the inner poverty which she unconsciously needed me to believe in. In analysis, she realized first of all that this internal poverty consisted of showing that she had a poor memory, a poor emotional life, and even poor health; but then she came to see that all these material and psychic riches of which she felt the need to be deprived, actually symbolized her sexual riches as a woman and hence were rooted in her body. This patient became giddy and faint whenever she displayed her riches, and above all when she showed me her feminine ability to take good care of her precious inner objects: she feared unconsciously that her mother, faced with the daughter's riches, might reproach her for being after the maternal wealth and wanting to get rid of a rival. It was as if she had told me, her transference-mother: 'Look here, I have nothing worth stealing, which proves that I have stolen nothing from you.'

For some female patients, presenting themselves as poor or miserable creatures reflects the need to show that they are not only incapable of taking care of their precious objects but that, moreover, they have none. 'For these patients, the ability to contain objects worth keeping by treating them in the best possible way, [is] a symbolic representation of the maternal genital organs which are capable of taking good care of the riches precious to the mother: the father's penis, embryos, and babies, and hence of containing them' (*ibid.*: 749).

In other cases, the symptom of apparent *poverty* may be closely related to, or sometimes coexist with, penis envy. The alarm signal sounds when the analysand fears that her apparent riches are not considered proof of her wish to have them taken for an equivalent of virility.

Emotional bisexuality in the two sexes

The study of competition-related vertigo in female analysands, with its various meanings according to whether it is linked more closely to their fear of having their female genitals amputated or to penis envy, demonstrates the influence of psychic bisexuality in women, and their ability to identify themselves with their mother as well as with their father.

This should alert us to the fact that the same phenomenon also appears in male analysands. To my mind, the most obvious interpretation of competition-related vertigo in men is the fear of surpassing the rival father, although envy of femininity sometimes occurs as well. That was why Luc was able to tell me that the vertigo which prevented him from climbing a ladder sometimes went with a feeling of faintness caused by the empty spaces between the rungs – so many hollows whose presence had been rendered 'objective'.

For Luc, these empty spaces proved to be a means of identifying himself with a female sex organ, which he had felt as posing an unconscious threat inasmuch as it might become revealed before he himself took cognizance of it in analysis.

------------------------------ 9 ------------------------------

Vertigo, from anxiety to pleasure

Every form of vertigo goes with a form of pleasure

Michael Balint (1959) has mentioned the 'thrills of pleasure' of those who enjoy the giddy sensation of fairground merry-go-rounds; these thrills recall the 'cries of joy' of the young child thrown up in the air and caught by his uncle to which Freud refers in *The Interpretation of Dreams* (1900a: 393). Can one and the same situation then cause anxiety as well as pleasure? On what conditions does either depend? The person who pays to go up in the big wheel at a fair knows what awaits him: why does he look forward to a dose of vertigo? Is it because he is certain that it will be no more than a dose and one moreover that, to some extent, serves to demystify the vertigo?

I believe that every form of vertigo goes with a particular form of pleasure. I shall give several examples of how an analysand can move from the anxiety pole towards the pleasure pole. In particular, I shall try to demonstrate that the pursuit of pleasure corresponding to each form of vertigo can be expressed in various types of sport. The reason why I have chosen sport as my example is the obvious physical connotation of the various manifestations of the symptom; but I might equally well have stressed that similar pleasures can be found in the arts, in professional work or in various leisure pursuits.

Pleasure and fusion-related vertigo: de-idealization of fusion

Enjoying fusion provided it can be dropped

A well-tempered fusion

Fusion-related vertigo goes hand in hand with the pleasure of feeling that one leads a life of one's own. In my opinion, one of the characteristics of this form of enjoyment lies paradoxically in the ability to experience fleeting moments of fusion. The reason why an analysand can grant himself moments of fusion is, on the one hand, that he has realized what riches fusion can provide in certain circumstances, and, on the other hand, that he is sufficiently aware of his own limits to allow him to emerge from the fusion: in fact, fusion proves useful and enriching provided it can be abandoned; it gives rise to vertigo if one believes one can never get out of it, but provides pleasure if one can savour it for brief moments.

It is only when fusion is idealized and desired as a permanent state that it becomes dangerous, because it is very hard to renounce what is considered a privileged relationship allowing one to cling to the object – so much so that anyone who has idealized fusion can see but two outcomes: either he plunges into it and runs the risk of becoming lost in it, or he flees from it and ends up in the void. Fusion idealized in this way holds a threat of vertigo no matter whether one succumbs to it or flees from it. Fusion must therefore have been de-idealized enough before moments of it can be accepted with pleasure: one must be absolutely certain of being able to get out of it and of recovering an object relationship.

Two everyday examples

Every one of us can, in various areas of his daily life, find experiences proving that the pleasure of living a separate existence can go hand in hand with moments of fusion: we might find it hard to fall asleep if we feared we might never wake up again, sleep being considered an experience of fusion in which the limits of one's ego are no longer perceptible; similarly, it is difficult to abandon oneself to orgasm if one is afraid that one may not be able to recover one's own dimensions. The pleasure of seeing a good film may also be considered a surrender to fusion: for two or three hours, the spectator can forget about being himself in his seat – he is up on the screen with the film's heroes. But in order to surrender to that fusion with the heroes, he must feel that when the lights go up again he will be brought back to himself. Some spectators are not sure of that, and if they do not want to miss seeing the film, they use such ruses as sitting close to the emergency light, which can help them to remember their identity at any given moment.

Perhaps it is in the intellectual field that the pleasure of feeling a distinct person has the most important consequences. To *comprehend* [*comprendre*] (that is, to *take into oneself* [lit.: *prendre avec*]) the other's thought, it is essential to experience a moment of fusion which consists of momentarily abandoning one's own form of thought in an attempt to follow the reasoning of the other. But that fusional step can only be taken if one can be sure of recovering one's own way of thinking afterwards. If one believes one will be unable to do that, one cannot make the least effort to understand the other. The pleasure of thinking springs from this game which facilitates, by successive fusions and defusions, the increasingly sharp definition of one's own thought and that of the other.

Positive moments of fusion in treatment

In the psychoanalysis of patients the de-idealization of fusion also plays an important role, because the analyst must not be afraid of experiencing moments of fusion with his analysands, especially when he agrees to treat patients who, at least at certain moments, use infraverbal modes of communication. For instance, when an analysand uses projective identification, unconsciously projecting into the analyst affects that enable the latter to test what the analysand was unable to convey to him verbally, the analyst must be able to accept this fusional approach instead of rejecting it for fear of losing his own affects. He needs to know that he can emerge from these moments of fusion in order to make use of them. It is then that the pleasure of feeling his separate existence can help the analyst, not to collude with his patient, but to find pleasure also in using this moment of fusion to arrive at a clearer differentiation. He can, for example, make positive use of the projective counter-identification described by Grinberg (1985).

In an article entitled 'Accepting fusion in order to emerge from it' (1991), J.-M. Quinodoz describes the case of a patient who complained of 'having no voice'. This symptom may or may not have had an organic basis, but it certainly had a psychic meaning: the patient suffered from a 'lack of self', that is, found it difficult to feel that she existed by herself, thought and felt by herself, which was reflected particularly in the difficulty she experienced in raising her own voice to make herself understood. She expected the analyst fused to her to speak for them both. J.-M. Quinodoz tells us how, after trying unsuccessfully to interpret the fusion and defusion, he decided to accept that the fusion was present in even the interpretative process, the better to shake it off; he then went on to interpret not using *I* or *you*, but *we*, thus reflecting the fusion of analyst and analysand. Here is an example of the interpretation he offered the patient when she complained of not having enough breath to speak: 'Everything happens as if we did not feel the difference between your breath and mine, between your respiration and mine, as if we had just one mouth between the two of us.' He went on to explain: 'Paradoxically enough, interpreting with the help of "we", far from strengthening the fusion in this aspect of our relationship, had an astonishing effect on the analysand; hearing me use "we" had the same effect on her as if she had been looking at herself in the mirror for the first time: after a moment of confusion, she realized that it was not a case of "we" but of her

103

and me, discovering as if for the first time that she had her own voice and that I had mine' (1991: 1699).

To benefit from the analysis, the analysand too must sometimes accept the fusion. In fact, the analysand suffering from fusion-related vertigo has very little freedom in his relationship with the analyst: he either desires fusion with the analyst or else he flees from it. It is only when he has rediscovered the possibility of emerging from fusion that he can risk becoming aware of the processes of introjection and projection in the transference, because he has become less afraid of losing his identity as a result.

'Interpretations in projection': an example of the positive use of fusion in psychoanalysis

Accepting 'well-tempered fusion' proves so helpful in some analyses that I should like to give an example of it. I propose to show, by *interpretations in projection*, how fusion can be used in psychoanalysis, provided it can be emerged from.

A useful interpretation with hard-to-reach analysands

The mute analysand's ego

By 'interpretations in projection' (D. Quinodoz 1994) I refer to a form of interpretation that proves useful with some analysands, and especially with those who, in a part of their ego, have a fusional relationship with an invasive internal object, corresponding most frequently to the introjection of a depressed, hypochondriac or suicidal parent. In some circumstances, or at certain points of the treatment, the analysand's ego may be too crushed or too overwhelmed by an object he has introjected, to hear what the analyst tells him. In particular, I have found that the part of some analysands' ego which had introjected an invasive object can itself become so invasive as to crush the rest of the ego, preventing it from exercising its critical faculty and from taking the analyst's interpretations into account. In fact, the confusion of the invading object with the part of the ego into which it has been introjected can lead the analysand to an unconscious adoption of the invading object's voice and way of feeling and thinking, as if they were his own. A patient may even, without realizing it, change his voice at certain moments of the treatment; if the analyst can make him aware of it, the patient may sometimes realize that he has unconsciously begun to speak like an important member of his family of whom he has rightly complained that he or she is invasive. If need be, this part of the ego can adopt the invasive attitude of the introjected object, tending to invade the rest of the ego.

It is precisely when he has the impression that the analysand's *real ego* has practically disappeared under the invasive object (or the part of the ego confused with the object) that the analyst may consider it useful to interpret in projection. By the analysand's *real ego* I refer to that part of his ego which has not been invaded by the introjected object, the part that has not been surrendered to the invader. It may well happen that the analysand's *real ego* has not disappeared, but that it has been projected into the analyst in an attempt to 'keep him safe from bad things inside' (one of the aims of projective identification listed by Hanna Segal (1973). In that case I think it very important for the analyst to be aware of the projection, to recognize the affects projected into him, and to agree to feel and verbalize them. The analysand will find his own feelings less frightening once he has come to realize that the analyst is able to feel, and to dare give a name to, what he, the patient, has rejected unconsciously because it does not conform to an object from which he could not bear to differentiate himself, lest he lose it or its love.

The analyst must therefore condone the fusion with the patient's ego projected into him, but only on condition that he can abandon it again! If he fails to do that, he would continue to collude with his patient and simply confirm the reality of the patient's phantasies.

The analyst as mouthpiece of the patient's ego

The most important phase in interpretation in projection involves the analyst in turning himself momentarily into the direct mouthpiece of the part of the analysand's ego projected into him, the analyst. The analyst then treats the comments of the analysand on the couch as if they came straight from the invasive introjected object, and not from the patient's ego, since the patient's *real ego* has been partly projected into the analyst. The analyst must take that projection into himself very seriously, agree to fuse with the patient's ego projected into him, treat very seriously the patient's fusion with the invasive object, and draw and interpret the consequences. In fact, the patient's *real ego*, as distinct from the invasive object, has been silenced because it has been projected into the analyst and hence can no longer be voiced through the patient's own mouth. To understand the feelings of the patient's true ego, the analyst must therefore act as their mouthpiece, and express directly what he feels the patient's ego projected into him might say if it could find the words. The analyst can then speak in the first person singular, using an 'I' that no longer refers to himself but to the part of the patient's ego projected into him. It is not enough for the analysand to realize that the feelings expressed by the analyst are *similar* to his own, which in this case might paradoxically threaten to strengthen the narcissistic illusion that analyst and analysand are alike. The analysand needs to become aware that these affects *are his* and emitted by the part of his ego projected into the analyst, which implies that analyst and analysand are two distinct, though related, objects.

In order to interpret in the projection, the analyst must recognize that the affects he has felt did not spring from him but from the analysand, and hence be keenly aware of what happens in the fusional relationship. That calls for the very special openness of the analyst described by Donald Meltzer: the analyst must be 'capable and willing, with regard to the observations and projections he receives . . . to submit the process to his unconscious . . . The analyst must . . . above all watch out for information from the very depths of his psyche about the emotional significance of the situation' (1984: 548). Of course, the analyst can be wrong and attribute to the patient what in reality comes from himself. We have had occasion to note that this is the risk every mother runs when she uses her capacity for reverie with her child.

An example of interpretation in projection

Marie is a young woman who was in analysis with me for a long time, attending for four sessions a week. After the first few months of analysis, she started an unbelievable phase of uninterrupted anger, which coincided with the announcement of my first vacation: she bombarded me with an incessant stream of insults and loud screams that grew worse from one session to the next. No matter whether I kept silent or interpreted the meaning of Marie's rage at the frustrating but appreciated object I represented for her (appreciated, because she continued to turn up regularly for her sessions), the volume and tone of her insults continued to swell in an auto-intoxicating crescendo that eventually became intolerable for me. I felt completely out of my depth, incapable of satisfying Marie, of calming her down or of discovering the meaning of her rage. I had the feeling that my words did not reach Marie's 'real' ego. On the other hand, when I listened to what went on in myself, I discovered a feeling of impotence as if before a tidal wave, and I said to myself: 'This is the all-invading sea (*mer*)'. In my counter-transference I noticed that I felt like a helpless little girl who is about to be crushed by an 'all-invading mother (*mère*)'.

It was then that I began to wonder if interpretation in the projection was called for. Was Marie, on the couch, not giving voice to a part of herself confused with an introjected object, the internal mother whom Marie felt to be invasive and never satisfied? An object that flung out her demands and her complaints through Marie's mouth? At the same time, didn't Marie project unconsciously into me her 'real' ego, that part of herself which, deprived of its natural rhythm and own needs, suffered from never being able to satisfy the invasive demands of a beloved mother?

That is why on hearing Marie say to me in a rage, 'It's now been months that I have been in analysis and I'm getting nowhere. Even if I waited for five hundred years you still wouldn't be doing anything!', I replied, 'Mummy always wants me to go faster; it's hard for me not to be able to keep my own little girl's pace'. Marie immediately calmed down, having recognized herself in my words. I said what her real ego was unable to feel and think; in effect, the only thing to speak through Marie's mouth was the exacting object that had invaded her. I later proffered her a complementary interpretation: 'Perhaps in reproaching me for not making haste, you were voicing what you imagine your mother might have said'. Marie then recovered that part of herself which she had projected into me and reintegrated it as her own. As a result she could abandon her confusion with the object, that is, with her mother, transferred in the analysis as confusion between her and me.

The analyst's containing function

The calming effect on Marie was connected not only to the reunification of her ego and to better understanding of the object whose invasive omnipotence seemed to have abated, but also to her discovery of the possible existence of an object relationship other than fusion or mutual invasion. This discovery, which had to be made time and again, was based on the experience of 'remaining oneself in one's relationship' with the analyst (Spira, 1985): Marie could recover what was hers as coming from herself, but now combined with the containing function of the analyst (as defined by Bion 1962), with which she could identify in order to contain herself. By means of the introjection of this containing function, the patient perceives the analyst as a good transference object; obviously there will also be other interpretations by which the analyst will present other aspects of the object in the transference, for instance the invasive object or the persecuting object.

Sport: the pleasure of fusion and differentiation

For some patients, sport is a means of giving physical expression, through their relationships with their surroundings, to the emotional work they do in order to play with their fusional desire and their wish to differentiate themselves from the object. Some patients, for instance, take pleasure in participating in such team sports as football, basketball or volleyball so as to feel in their bodies the constant see-saw motion between the identity of the team and that of the individual player. It is the team that wins or loses, but only thanks to the action or mistake of a given player. A great deal of work is involved in fusion with the team, which only becomes possible if the player maintains his personal identity, and if he can, for example, not break down when his team loses. Other analysands may try to seek to externalize their inner work of defusion and differentiation through physical experience involving not a team but a more cosmic object. They take pleasure in becoming aware of their bodies by practising such techniques as yoga or doing certain physical exercises that render them more attentive to the process involved in differentiating themselves physically from what is not their own self.

Clearly, in the practice of one and the same sport, different patients introduce different aspects of the quest for pleasure: in the same sport, some will find physical pleasure in well-tempered fusion, while others may find it in the psychic effort involved in competition. I shall not recall this diversity in every form of pleasure I shall be discussing, but shall merely look at several sports particularly characteristic of the pleasure that can accompany them.

Pleasure and vertigo related to being dropped: de-idealization of the carrying object

The pleasure corresponding to vertigo related to being dropped strikes me as being connected with the de-idealization of the containing or carrying object. In effect, for patients who have analysed their vertigo related to being dropped, the containing or carrying object is no longer omnipotent or held to be solely responsible for containing or carrying them, be it only because they have come to appreciate the active part they themselves play in the constitution of the object and in the attitude the object adopts. Paradoxically, the fear of being dropped by the object can go hand in hand with the pleasure of allowing oneself measured *doses of being dropped by it*. That pleasure depends on the feeling that the dropping is not irreversible and definite, but that it is a positive process of separation and reunion. Every one of us has been able to witness the surprise of a small child who discovers that he can take – previously unthinkable – pleasure in leaving his mother to go to school or to visit a playmate, knowing that she will still be there when he comes back.

The chance presence of a free object favoured over the certain presence of a controlled object

These analysands may, for instance, set about choosing their surroundings with great care instead of putting up with things as they are, or merely complaining about them. They dare to look at the differences between objects and, as far as possible, try to surround themselves with objects with which they can feel confident and free, and no longer constrained or passive. We might add that these analysands then make a point of spending time on choosing their partners in various spheres of life: for instance, a salaried analysand may put in as much care in choosing his employer as an employer does in choosing his staff, or a housewife in choosing her domestic help; they do the same when it comes to their social partners or lovers, instead of allowing themselves to be at the whim of chance and leaving it until it is too late to discover whether the partner suits them or not. An important criterion for choosing one's partner is then to ascertain whether relations can be established with them on a basis of mutual trust, which implies freedom, and not on the basis of suspicion, which implies controlling everything and demanding accountability. The priority accorded to this criterion implies preferring 'losing the security afforded by the assured presence of the controlled object in order to gain the quality of presence of a free object' (D. Quinodoz 1994: 760).

Let me mention the case of one of my analysands who could not refrain from telephoning me during the sessions he missed, even when he had told me beforehand about his absence; he was ashamed to do so, but he simply had to make sure that I had not given his place to someone else. He no longer had a need to do that the day he became aware of the role he had assigned to me in the transference: that of a parent whom he could not trust, one who was only too ready to take a greater interest in somebody else the moment the analysand took his eyes off him. The patient had now come to appreciate that he was entitled to make distinctions between objects, that while it was naive not to check up on some people, it was quite ridiculous not to trust others. However, he knew what he was giving up when he surrounded himself with trustworthy objects: 'When you are away and I feel confident that I am important to you, then I know perfectly well that you will come to find me as soon as you can; I shall be calm, but you will be away all the same and I shall suffer from your absence. On the other hand, if I do not feel confident in you, I can tie you down, and there are many ways of doing that, and then I can be sure that you stay here. Being sure of your presence is an advantage, but actually that advantage is worthless because you would be kept here by force and I am no longer interested in that.'

Taking care of one's important objects

Another new attitude results from the fact that these analysands have come to appreciate the active part played by their ego in the construction of the internal object; they now begin to take good care of their important objects because they realize that there is an interaction between their way of treating the object and its smooth functioning; they feel that the object is sensitive and vulnerable and hence needs to be properly tended if it is to behave well.

These analysands also discover the idea of psychic well-being; a taste for treating themselves well and for treating the other well becomes an important acquisition. That taste often involves a concern for external well-being considered as a prerequisite of optimum functioning and hence providing the pleasure that goes with doing one's best. Thus it is often after the analysis of vertigo related to being dropped that analysands realize how astonished they were at my attention to our mutual convenience involved in, say, agreeing a timetable during the preliminary interviews, because they themselves would never have dared to attach any importance to the matter.

Sport: the pleasure of being dropped and carried

I have been describing a quest for pleasure by which the analysand tries to establish good container–contained relationships with his internal objects. This quest can sometimes take the form of a physical pleasure externalizing, in the patient's relations with his surroundings, what happens in his relations with his internal objects. We can see this in the pleasure analysands can take in certain activities in which the sportsman plays with the pleasure of administering measured 'doses of being dropped' to himself. The most typical example is probably parachuting, a pursuit in which the parachutist gives himself the pleasure of being dropped without having to fear a disaster; this may possibly also explain the passion for bungee jumping. I believe that sports such as hang-gliding, para-gliding or gliding are further typical examples of sports in which the sportsman can try to establish good relations with an object by doing all he can to turn it into a good container or carrier. Without the action of the sportsman who takes good care of his hang-glider or para-glider and knows how to use it properly, these devices would be of small use as carriers; to add to the thrill, there is the ever-present chance of a mishap. But other sports, such as skiing, surfing, mountaineering and even swimming can also be held in high regard by sportsmen playing this kind of game with the container–contained relationship. Thus the swimmer may be specially interested to do all he can to make the water carry him efficiently, and appreciates that it is in his own power to render his relationship with the water more effective.

Pleasure and suction-related vertigo: de-idealization of the imprisoning object

Here we find the same mechanism as we met in the last example: the object loses its omnipotence when the analysand discovers his own active role in its construction, and especially in its tendency to suck in or imprison. As a result, his new attitudes strike me as being congruent with those associated with the pleasure described in connection with vertigo related to being dropped. The pleasure of not allowing oneself to be imprisoned by the internal object can be externalized and be given physical expression through certain sports. We have seen that swimming may be liked above all for the pleasure it provides in turning the water into a *carrier*, but it can also appeal because of the pleasure of feeling oneself sucked in by the sea or its contents, in the full knowledge that the resulting imprisonment is temporary and can be kept under control. Some sports seem particularly appropriate to express-ing this form of pleasure, among them deep-sea diving and speleology; however, even these sports can reflect other forms of searching for pleasure or several forms at once, and their popularity is constantly changing.

Pleasure and imprisonment/escape-related vertigo: de-idealization of immutability and change

Alternation becomes integration into the psychic world

When a patient tries, in action, to satisfy contrary intentions without com-bining them, he can only do so one at a time. By contrast, in psychic life contrary trends can coexist: we can phantasize opposite scenarios, but above all we can be moved at one and the same time by different or even opposite feelings within us. I cannot at one and the same time run away from prison and run back to it – it is one or the other. By contrast, I can at one and the same time have the wish to escape from, and to be locked up in, a prison. The anxiety consequent upon experiencing contrary trends within oneself corresponds to the pleasure of giving oneself measured doses of that experience.

Inasmuch as this ambivalence is experienced in linear, chronological order, it can trigger off vertiginous anxiety and immobilize those who experience it. By contrast, when it is experienced in the representative context of a personal history constantly altered, that is, in the context of a mental world occupying space and time, this ambivalence can give those who experience it the impres-sion that they are involved in a constantly fresh process of creation and thus convey a feeling of deep inner riches. The affective currents no longer move along a single line of force, where they can only be added together, subtracted

111

from one another or cancelled out, but in multi-dimensional space where their combination produces a resultant and a new direction. This is tantamount to the awareness that the internal world is vast, that it can contain an infinity of feelings capable of combining and modifying one another. At any one moment, their result is an original and irreplaceable creation, characteristic of the analysand and affording him deep pleasure.

There are some sports that exemplify this quest for the pleasure of combining contradictory feelings and wishes. As always, these sports can of course also be chosen for other reasons; in any case some sportsmen delight particularly in the contrast between being imprisoned in the cramped space of a boat, of a glider or a racing car and the freedom to roam the immensity of the ocean, of the sky or the roads. Thus a journalist who interviewed Bertrand Piccard, after his crossing of the Atlantic in a balloon in September 1992, asked him if it had not been a very trying experience for two people to be enclosed for several days in so small a space, was told by Piccard that it would have been even more trying to get out: 'Of course, we were enclosed in a space of four square metres, but our capsule was more crammed with dreams than anyone can imagine'. That capsule was both tiny and yet without limits and that constituted its charm, something for which Piccard was ready to put up with a great deal of inconvenience.

This is also what some analysands and analysts appreciate about psychoanalysis: the analyst's room can seem very small for two people to meet in several times a week for many years, but it opens up on the immensity of the psyche, of the unconscious, of duration, of the mystery that is enshrined in every person; for some people this constitutes the profound charm of an adventure for which they are ready to suffer what are sometimes very painful moments.

Alternation becomes integration over time; there is no longer the least conflict between the continuity of the object and its ability to change

What the analysand discovers in all this toing and froing into and out of prison is that the subject and the object, developing in psychic space and time, are at the meeting point of the continuous and the discontinuous. What we have here is therefore a search for a pleasurable experience resulting from the combination of the continuous, unchangeable aspect of the object and its discontinuous and changing aspect.

Patients prone to imprisonment/escape-related vertigo express a form of anxiety arising from changes in the analyst no less than from his continuity. Faced with changes in the analyst, these patients complain that they cannot trust an object that alters, and note all changes in the analyst's physical appearance or dress, or all changes in his rooms, which are often considered extensions of the analyst's personality: 'Whom can I trust if even my analyst changes? I ought to be able to count on you!' said one patient one day when I had changed the arrangement of the paintings in the waiting room. This patient was always afraid of our separations because he was sure that they made me change and that he might not recognize me again – that, on his next visit, he would be faced with a different, unknown object. Change, seen as proof of the object's discontinuity, generated a need for an immutable object.

And yet this same patient objected to the boredom produced by an immutable object, and what he feared most of all was that the analysis might become monotonous one day, making him wish to run away. That patient mistook the absence of change in the object for its constancy, so much so that he turned the absence of change in the object into a criterion of its reliability. As a result, the reliable and constant object, supposed never to change, became a boring prison from which the patient was keen to escape. He had reached an impasse: if the object was to cease being a boring prison it had to change, but such change struck him as being a source of insecurity – once the object could change it could no longer be relied upon.

This vertiginous coming and going between the desire for a continuous and immutable object and the longing for a changing and discontinuous object turned into a search for dynamic pleasure once this patient had integrated continuity and change; that is, once he had realized that an object could undergo changes and yet remain constant and reliable. Change had become development; there was no longer the least incompatibility between continuity and change.

Patients open to this aspect of the search for integration of the continuous and the discontinuous, of the changeable and the immutable, express their quest for pleasure by taking a special interest in every sport that plays with transformations of the object: there are skiers, for example, who pay special attention to changes in the quality of the snow during the course of the day; they take pleasure in returning to the same ski resort because part of their pleasure is tied up with noticing changes in their way of skiing on one and the same piste, depending on changes in the quality of the snow. These patients are also extremely fond of such sports as ice-skating which depends on an object, the ice, whose ephemeral make-up is bound up with a point of equilibrium: the quality of the ice changes with the temperature, but above a certain threshold the ice disappears: the object is constant despite changes in temperature to a certain point, but above that point the object becomes unrecognizable and disappears. Great sportsmen can play with the continuity and the discontinuity of the object, even when engaged in sports that strike the uninitiated as being devoid of that aspect: thus when running or long-jump champions evaluate their performances, they take the speed and direction of the wind into account.

113

Pleasure and vertigo related to attraction to the void: de-idealization of the void and of projection

Pleasure and the active form of vertigo related to attraction to the void

The active form of this vertigo is characterized on the one hand by the projection into empty space of drives, that is, of needs and wishes of which the analysand hopes unconsciously to rid himself, and on the other hand by the wish to repossess these projections. The resulting anxiety is complex and its various forms are interrelated: at one and the same time the analysand feels anxious about his own drives, which leads him to expel them; about the impoverishment and inner void caused by these expulsions; about the external void as the projection of the intolerable inner void; and about his overwhelming desire to fling himself into the external void to recover what he has expelled into it. To each of these anxieties corresponds the pleasure of surmounting it; to each of these forms of vertigo corresponds the pleasure of taking a measured dose of what in a different context would have caused anxiety.

De-idealizing the omnipotence of the drives

Once the drive has lost its magical power, analysands have less need to expel it; they are brave enough to re-appropriate it instead. They can allow themselves moments in which they play at expelling and re-appropriating their libidinal and aggressive drives.

Some analysands can express the re-appropriation of their aggressive drives by taking up more or less violent sports either individually, for instance in judo, karate or boxing, or as part of a team, for instance in rugby or American football. Others again can express the re-appropriation of their libidinal impulses by taking pleasure in their prowess at certain sports that may be unconscious and successful sublimations of their sexual prowess. I am thinking particularly of acrobats, working by themselves or in couples, and of people participating in gymnastic displays or in figure skating. But in fact this process extends to all analysands who enjoy feeling that their bodies are working smoothly, or discovering what improves their physical prowess.

De-idealization of projection

One way of overcoming the anxiety about the void created by one's projections is expecting to recoup them. This can be done once the analysand has lost his belief in the omnipotence of projection: the object no longer has the magical

114

power of retaining the projections, and the subject can therefore keep in touch with his own projections. One way in which he can do that may be by taking care of the object into which they have been projected. Thus while there are many ways of engaging in equestrian sports, for some people riding or taking care of a horse can be an unconscious means of taking good care of themselves through the horse, and/or of allowing themselves to experience, through the horse, impulses they do not allow themselves to experience directly.

De-idealization of the object that receives the projections

The analysand who hopes to rid himself forever of his projections may succumb to vertigo at the very thought of trying to recover them. But the vertigo makes way for pleasure once he begins to realize that there are interactions and a dependent relationship between the person who projects and the one who receives the projections. He discovers the pleasure of enjoying the mobility of subject and object, and of their relationship, even in their continuity. We find that pleasure in all forms of sports involving the training and taming of animals, even though these sports may sometimes give expression to other facets of the personality.

The de-idealization of the internal void

Here we come to a characteristic aspect of the pleasure corresponding to the active form of vertigo related to attraction to the void. It reflects the analysand's anxiety about feeling empty inside, a feeling he often created by the expulsion of what he dreaded in himself, thus turning his internal void into an external one. The de-idealization of the internal void, by robbing it of its magical omnipotence, allows the analysand to take pleasure in allowing himself to be attracted to this internal void (which is at the origin of the attracting external void), because he guesses that what he had taken for a void may, in fact, be a psychic space left for him to discover. An analysand who had been complaining about his inner void for a long time declared, after a silence in an analytic session, 'The reason why I am keeping silent today is not that I feel empty, but that I feel an inner silence'. That day, she was no longer afraid of her internal void – it had become inhabited.

De-idealization of the 'black hole'

An analysand may sometimes find this pleasure directly in the analytic work: this is true above all of analysands whose vertigo is accompanied by

115

terrifying phantasies of falling into a black hole (D. Quinodoz 1996) and who, like the characters in Patrick Modiano's novels, have the feeling that their life, albeit highly complex in appearance, is actually built on a hole and lacks foundations and roots. They have terrifying spells of vertigo because everything of interest they can experience, be it good or bad, threatens to slip into that hole, leaving them with nothing.

These patients give the analyst clearly to understand how much, in their vertigo, atrocious anxiety can go hand in hand with a search for pleasure. In fact, at the beginning of their analysis, and then at certain moments during its later course, they panic at the very idea of looking with the analyst at anything resembling that phantasy hole. They want above all to shut their eyes to it; the analyst knows perfectly well that the most likely reason why they have constructed this phantasy hole under their internal house, was to hide monsters even more terrifying than the void. Yet the realization that the black hole is not a void but filled with riches is an essential step for the analysand, inasmuch as there is a crucial difference between feeling that one has originated from *nothing* (in which case one has the impression of having been *nothing* from the outset, of not having sprung from the primal scene: one's whole self would have been created by the environment after the event), and feeling that one has sprung from a badly organized but rich *original chaos*, capable of making sense and of giving rise to life (because one has the feeling of having been rich from the outset, even if it is not easy to organize these explosive riches and to combine them with the contributions of the environment).

The analysand's vertigo can become transformed into 'thrills of pleasure' as soon as, jointly with the analyst, he dares to look into the basement of his life and comes to appreciate that the monsters he projected and believed unconsciously to be about to leap out are perhaps less dangerous than he imagined. I say jointly, because the analysand cannot get rid of his defence mechanism – the creation of a void in phantasy – unaided, the monsters being too terrifying to face by someone still lacking solid foundations. The transformation of panic into pleasure does not happen without much toing and froing; it takes a great deal of courage for the analysand to dare look into the black hole, especially when the building erected on top of it seems highly elaborate and attractive and holds out the promise of shelter much like a mobile home that has no need of foundations. But this shelter does not last, and at the first difficulty the analysand has the impression that everything is about to slip back into the void. It is worth noting that there is a stage allowing the analysand to take fresh courage during his joint exploration with the analyst: namely the appearance of the idea of a *trap-door*. If the analysand wishes to, he can discover the initial hole by opening the trap door, while, by closing the trap door, he can build foundations ensuring that all the contents are not dissipated into the void. The trap-door concept allows the analysand to toy with his fascination with, and his horror of, the internal void.

I have been struck by the fact that patients suffering from such vertiginous 'black holes' need the analyst to provide them with representations; they cannot reconstruct their foundations and their basement unless they are provided with mental images that enable them to experience bodily sensations corresponding to what they construct psychically and symbolically. I believe that what they have been missing for the construction of the emotional 'basement' of their bodily ego was something so early that, in order to rediscover it in analysis, they needed to re-experience the basic physical sensations involved in the elaboration of their thought at the start of their lives. The interpretations must accordingly be full of references to colour, sound, smell and touch; this fact has enabled me to appreciate what can be so particularly fascinating in non-figurative art for those to whom such paintings recall the ineffable nature of the first sensations underlying the beginnings of the first thoughts.

A dream mentioned by Anny Duperey in her *Le voile noir* might serve as an illustration of the ambivalent feeling composed of anxiety and pleasure that some people experience at the idea of exploring the basement of their internal house; her image of the house may be considered a representation of the author herself or of her personal history. In fact, in the elaboration of her own history, Anny Duperey was hampered by the absence of any memory of her early childhood before the violent death of her parents: she had simply forgotten them. The reconstruction of her history was accordingly like a house whose basement or cellar she did not know. In recounting her dream, she reveals her unconscious ambivalence about growing or not growing flowers in the subsoil of her house. She portrays that ambivalence by means of a subtle game in which, as a dreamer, she considers that her wish to take care of the cellar and to make it flower is really her own, while her wish to let it fall into decay is something she does not recognize as her own and hence attributes to others, that is, to her family. Here I can only quote fragments of this dream and would refer the reader to the full text, which alone can convey the richness of this book:

> And I went right down to the bottom, where, in the half light, I could only just make out a part of the soil already cultivated, and my spade sank as if into butter . . . During this time, the voice of the others, outside, became more and more urgent in their attempts to discourage me . . . And I went to the door, mounted a few steps, spade in hand, to persuade them not to do so – that, yes, things would grow nicely down there, you will see! And turning back, I discovered at the same time as they did a marvellous multi-coloured carpet of flowers that had sprung up all by itself . . . I had made flowers grow in a cellar . . .
>
> (1992: 187–8)

To appreciate that the two wishes, to cultivate and not to cultivate her cellar, were both the dreamer's own, we must not forget that in the dream, created by the dreamer in her sleep, all the elements came from the dreamer herself: she herself had invented the entire scenario, even the feelings and desires she attributed to others. It was indeed Anny Duperey the dreamer who had imagined in her dream that flowers could grow in her cellar, but who had also imagined that they could not; by attributing the second of these phantasies to others, she disowned them in a way, yet demonstrated her ambivalence: her anxiety and pleasure at the idea of digging in the sub-soil of her personal history.

Internal void or inner silence?

The anxiety associated with vertigo related to attraction to the void para-doxically goes hand in hand with the pleasure of granting oneself brief experiences of an inner void; that pleasure appears the moment the internal void assumes a meaning, even if that meaning is still unconscious, at a time when the void cannot really be called 'empty'. I have been amazed to dis-cover analysands who begin to grant themselves momentary glimpses of an *internal void* without knowing what pleasures awaited them there; sometimes they even seemed rather ashamed as if these were wasted moments or shameful satisfactions. Depending on their character, they gave different names to these moments: moments of silence, of meditation, of withdrawal, of not thinking, of dozing, of solitude. It is often later in the analysis that they come to realize how valuable these moments were, facilitating as they did psychic activity in a new mode and rhythm.

With these analysands, these moments of experiencing an *internal void* are sometimes a reason for indulging in leisure activities that, at first sight, seem surprising because it is hard to see what pleasure they provide. One might say to oneself, 'Walking for hours and hours, even if the countryside is beau-tiful, what masochism!' or 'Doing interminable lengths in a swimming pool, what a mindless thing to do!' or, again, 'Mowing the lawn, how boring!' One might think the same thing of all leisure activities involving repetitive actions. In fact, if we leave aside athletic training, the reason why some analysands take to these leisure activities is often that the repetitive rhythm helps them to find, not an internal void, but the pleasure of inner silence. Of course, I am only referring to repetitive activities chosen freely by these patients. Some do not need this repetitive activity to grant them-selves the delight of moments of inner silence; they can, for instance, find it through art, or again by adopting an inner listening attitude; every one of us must discover his own way by himself.

One of the privileged ways of discovering the pleasure of inner silence is undoubtedly analysis itself. Many patients feel anxious, at the beginning of their analysis, about indulging four times a week in these periods of inner silence, for which they nevertheless feel the need intuitively. 'I shall have nothing to say!', 'All this wasted time!', 'Staring at my navel all this time!' they keep complaining. True, rationally considered, in our civilization in which the pursuit of efficiency is held in such high regard, this apparent waste of time does seem sterile, or at least counter-productive. But, more often, the analysand who discovers the riches of his inner world and who originally felt that he had nothing useful to say, also discovers the importance of what seems to be so useless. Actually, the reason why the inner silence is gradually felt to be precious by some analysands is that it facilitates closer listening not only to their own inner world but also to the inner worlds of persons important to them; they then have the feeling of opening themselves up to a previously unsuspected space.

I believe that this discovery of the inner silence in analysis is largely bound up with the joint presence of two factors: on the one hand the large number of weekly analytic sessions (my analysands generally attend four times a week) and their regularity, and on the other hand the way of listening – sometimes called 'silent' – adopted by the analyst. While the frequency and regularity of the sessions create a repetitive rhythm that encourages the emergence of the analysand's inner silence, the analyst's *silence* renders the analysand attentive to his inner world, because this particular silence is not a form of keeping quiet but of listening to everything the analysand brings up; in fact, the analyst does not hesitate to speak whenever he feels that this may encourage the emergence of the patient's psychic reality and his listening to his own inner world. I believe that the analyst is led to create a silence within himself by which what is internal can make itself heard. It is in this sense that I understand the following passage by André Green:

> The silent function of the analyst is independent of the number of words (or information) he introduces into the analytic setting. In fact, this function depends on the silence the analyst keeps in his interpretative response to the manifest content of the discourse.
>
> (1980: 8)

Listening to their inner world enables some analysands to discover within themselves an affective richness whose existence they never suspected, and if they should then succeed in verbalizing it they will discover a host of ever more interesting nuances. One of my analysands, a keen sportsman, told me with great surprise: 'I once told my wife that I loved her and since she then knew that I did, I saw no point in repeating it. What's more I stopped thinking about it. And then, in analysis, I thought about it again and I told her once more, and then it was as if I had rediscovered what I had felt. I never imagined that feelings were like muscles, that they need to be exercised to keep in shape, and in order to exercise them they have to be put into words.' I shall not dwell on possible transferential interpretations of that phrase, but merely point out the discovery by this analysand and the physical references it elicited: for these affects to come into life, he had to verbalize them, to repeat them time and again, or risk their atrophy.

Pleasure and the passive form of vertigo related to attraction to the void: de-idealization of the magical void

The passive form of vertigo related to attraction to the void involves the fear of being drawn into unfathomable outer depths – air, water or even the earth; of being engulfed and disappearing for ever. When the analysand de-idealizes the unfathomable void, it loses its magical omnipotence; the void becomes a space and begins to assume boundaries and a shape, and to obey laws we can learn about and come to understand. The analysand will then take great pleasure in leaping into the void, knowing that he will find a space in it. Some analysands actually derive pleasure from advancing into external space, even while realizing that they cannot always tell its boundaries, but knowing fully well that there are some. They then discover enough signposts to make them lose the fear that this external space has an unlimited and magical attractive power, one that cannot be explained and that obeys no laws.

Localizing the absence of a bottom

The phantasy underlying this form of vertigo related to attraction to the void is very widespread, and I have often found that patients need to reassure themselves by means of this phantasy that there is a specific place where the sky and the sea are without a bottom and threaten to suck them into infinity.

One attempt to derive pleasure from this anxiety may involve looking for a bottom in the external world, rather than going in fear of being sucked in by the universe at large; the immediate satisfaction is the realization that there is no longer a reason for avoiding air or sea travel, since all the traveller need do to banish the anxiety is to avoid these suction holes; this defence against anxiety is well known because it corresponds to the classic mechanism of phobia. Such natural phenomena as the Bermuda Triangle or the bottom of Loch Ness arouse the particular interest of patients suffering from this type of vertigo; but their interest is reinforced above all by a phantasy that enthrals them and that is related to their vertiginous fear of being sucked into a bottomless universe: namely the phantasy of pinpointing in, say, the Bermuda Triangle or the unfathomable bottom of Loch Ness, the hole in the universe into which they can be sucked to disappear for ever in a mysterious beyond that has even ceased to be the universe.

Another attempt to find pleasure by pinpointing the phantasy hole in the universe seems to me to be the imaginary creation of a monster as the positive counterpart of what the hole conjures up negatively; the terrifying aspects of this phantasy hole are not its edges, which are positive and open to representation, but the empty parts which are negative and cannot be represented. The Loch Ness monster, for instance, might be a representation of the frightening hole through which the lake could suck one in: it is much easier to struggle against an anxiety that has a name or a face, especially if that face is represented as being as inoffensive as it is frightening. I believe that the popular fascination with the 'abominable snowman' reflects the same type of defence mechanism against the anxiety of being sucked in by a magical hole in the universe, localized in the impassable Himalayas, through which anyone venturing to go would disappear from the universe for ever.

The projection of a void replaced with that of a welcoming space

Another quest for pleasure involves a deeper change in the patient's relations with his internal objects. In fact, the reason why I dwell on the phantasy underlying this form of vertigo is that the more the patient suffers from the passive form of suction-related vertigo, the more he projects the picture of a female genital hole which can hold nothing and in which everything disappears, into the universe; whereas the closer the patient draws to the pleasure pole, the more he projects onto the outside hollow, structured and accommodating female genitals. Obviously, the patient might equally well phantasize that he is in danger of disappearing into a universe perceived as a hollow female sex organ clinging aggressively to its content. But on the one hand, this dread of a more highly structured swallowing object is less frightening than the fear of an amorphous swallowing object, because the patient knows at least where the aggressor is hiding and what defensive action he must take; and on the other hand, inasmuch as the swallowing object is more clearly defined, vertigo related to attraction to the void makes way for suction-related vertigo.

This pleasure of penetrating into a space that has ceased to be a magical aspirator, of exploring it and of discovering landmarks in it, includes the pleasure of allowing oneself to be sucked into, or to be briefly fascinated by, that space, knowing that these landmarks are there so that it is possible to find one's way out again. This pleasure of measuring up to a welcoming space is close to the pleasure of genital penetration, but experienced on the symbolic plane. That particular quest for pleasure may involve physical participation as happens with all those who, from para-gliders to astronauts, penetrate physically into space, a universe they delight in exploring; others again, for instance speleologists or volcanologists, prefer to penetrate the bowels of the earth; while yet others like to probe the depths of the ocean. All of them have the feeling that despite everything – and this strikes me as being part of their pleasure – the limits of the ocean, of the sky or of the earth are far away and mysterious and that they run some risk of being swallowed up in them; yet what makes for pleasure is the fact that the danger is no longer magical and that by keeping carefully to certain rules, the delights of penetration outweigh the threat of being engulfed. The pleasure of penetrating into the unfathomable universe can also be purely psychic, as in the case of the astronomer who penetrates the sky with the help of his telescopes.

The analysand discovers the pleasure of a permissible form of secondary curiosity: the curiosity of seeing, of knowing, of learning how that space is constituted now that it is no longer magical. This is a form of psychic curiosity, the right to know what the world is made of, what one's mother's body is made of, to understand the mechanics of sexual life; but a curiosity that can be expressed in many different ways, from enjoying the pleasure of satisfying one's scientific curiosity and daring to reveal one's discoveries, through allowing oneself the phantasies of an artist's curiosity and daring to exhibit one's creations, down to the pleasure of exploring caves, the ocean bed, virgin territory, or sailing the Atlantic solo. This pleasure can also be enjoyed by the psychoanalyst who tries to penetrate the depths of the unconscious in order to discover landmarks that will keep him from disappearing into it.

Pleasure and expansion-related vertigo: de-idealization of ego-expansion

Ego-expansion clashes with object expansion

As we have seen, expansion-related vertigo is perceived by analysands wishing to push back the limits of their ego incessantly, in the hope that this continuous expansion will afford them a keener sense of existence, but feeling at the same time that if this idealized expansion does not come up against any limits put up by the objects, it will be transformed into narcissistic haemorrhage and a loss of identity.

Analysands begin to take pleasure when, ceasing to accord such omnipotence to the expansion of their ego, they can allow themselves to experience moments of an ego expansion that no longer threatens to turn into narcissistic haemorrhage: their vertigo disappears and makes way for positive narcissistic pleasure once they feel that they can momentarily give way to an expansion of their ego and then resume listening to others. At the end of his analysis, Yves, whom I have mentioned in connection with this form of vertigo, began to take intense pleasure in putting his point of view across at lectures, just as soon as he felt capable of stopping his ego expansion at the end of his address to take in the views of others and to measure his limits up against theirs. He thus recovered his feeling of being himself in the pleasure of an expansion that was permissible because it was under his control.

Pleasure of ego expansion expressed through sport

I believe that this desire to push oneself as far as possible, until one feels that one has reached the absolute limit, that is the point where the expansion stops, corresponds to attempts by sportsmen to achieve the impossible. In sport, they feel intense pleasure in extending their limits as far as they possibly can, to where narcissistic haemorrhage begins. I am thinking of such famous skiers as Sylvain Saudan, of divers who dispense with aqualungs, trying to plumb their physiological limits, or of solitary sailors and explorers who push their own limits as far as possible while braving solitude as a measure of their physical condition, and also of explorers who take pleasure in discovering how far they can go in extending their knowledge of themselves and of the Other, the unknown.

Pleasure and competition-related vertigo: de-idealization of victory

Patients liable to competition-related vertigo are caught in a conflict between their longing for omnipotent victory over their rivals and castration anxiety. Since vertigo prevents the victory, it helps them avoid the threat of castration. In fact, it is only when a patient idealizes victory that the conflict becomes intolerable so that the risks entailed by victory must be nipped in the bud with the help of vertigo. During spells of vertigo, the patient imagines himself eternally victorious over his rival, whom he has crushed for good. The pleasure corresponding to competition-related vertigo involves a paradox once again: the patient begins to take pleasure in allowing himself victories because he has de-idealized them.

De-idealization of victory over time

Some analysands cannot allow themselves to succeed because, having idealized success, they are afraid that it may freeze time in an eternal triumph:

there is no longer any *afterwards* and success becomes synonymous with death; in order to finish a task they have begun (studies, theses, constructions, etc.) they must feel certain that something else can be expected to follow. When these patients begin to de-idealize victory over time, they grant themselves the pleasure of trying for success because such success will be part of an ongoing story and will leave them a loophole: winning today does not necessarily mean winning tomorrow. Pleasure then appears because success no longer freezes time magically but allows an 'afterwards'.

On the whole, it is unusual for a sportsman to be content with remaining at the level he has reached; he is constantly trying to do better and to make further progress. This is in keeping with what we know about equilibrium which, be it psychic or physical, is never secured but must be constantly re-established. We know that someone who does not progress in a sport runs the risk of losing ground, and that those who believe they have established so good a relationship with an important object that they no longer need to take care of it are well on the way to losing it.

De-idealization of victory by extension

Patients may also de-idealize victory extensively: I win in one field but in others my rival can be allowed to be better than I am. This allows these patients to accept victory because it leaves them with a way out. Thus I can permit myself to climb higher than my father in the professional field, because I think the world of what he does in some other sphere. It is extremely common that, during their analysis, patients suffering from this type of vertigo discover areas in which, to their great surprise, they have always admired their father without realizing it.

De-idealization of victory by phantasy games

It is true that some scenarios seem to be the very opposite of the one I have just described. Thus, during very high-level competitions, some sportsmen can be heard to address extremely violent remarks to their opponents. Before the match, a distinguished sportsman may look down on his opponent as so much dirt and promise himself to grind him into dust to teach him a lesson once and for all. I wonder if what we have here may not be another way of de-idealizing the aggressive omnipotence of the rivalry: by accepting an imaginary scenario in which all the hatred of his rival can be expressed in phantasy, the sportsman saves himself the trouble of killing his oedipal rival in reality, but also of having to loathe him for ever.

A sportsman can play this drama, in phantasy, at different – especially pre-

or post-oedipal – levels. In other words, some sportsmen take pleasure, in phantasy, in playing the Oedipus drama before it has been resolved: they delight in killing their father in their phantasy at every match or tournament, and they enjoy that pleasure precisely because in phantasy everything is allowed. Others again enact the Oedipus drama, still in the course of elaboration or even fully elaborated, in competitions, because they prefer the pleasure of fighting the rival to that of killing him.

De-idealization of the rivals' presence

Another way of finding pleasure in rivalry can take the form of de-idealizing the winner's position: space is vast, there is not just one winning run, there are as many as there are rivals and moreover everybody is his own rival. 'All the better if my father climbs to the top of his ladder; I have a ladder of my own. The important thing for me is to beat my own record and to reach the top of *my* ladder.' These patients do not normally play a lot of competitive games, and if they do after their vertigo has been cured, and perhaps come out as winners, they do so for the pleasure of bettering their own performance, not for the pleasure of outdoing others.

De-idealization of the magic of victory

This particular de-idealization proved to be one of the most important for Luc. At the beginning of his analysis, he could not permit himself any professional success, because he always felt that he had stolen it. For a long time, he could not rid himself of the impression that, if he showed the results of his professional research to his colleagues, or worse still to his employers, he would be frowned upon; hence he never explained how he had arrived at his results – it was as if he had come by them through magic. Not only did he not sign his work, but on several occasions, forced to explain it verbally, he was seized by attacks of vertigo so intense that he had to ask a colleague to take his place.

All this was in sharp contrast with the pleasure he took, at the end of his analysis, in explaining to his colleagues in detail how he had arrived at his conclusions; moreover, one of the characteristics of his presentations, on which he was congratulated, was to show how he had learned, from his mistakes and failures, to improve his work, finding better answers every time he did so. He could at long last allow himself to take pleasure in his successes because he had not reached them by magic but had researched hard to obtain them – they were his own. This made me think of some artists at the peak of their fame; they told admirers who asked them how

125

they had managed to produce such masterpieces: 'By working hard at them'. True, that does not explain their creations, but it does justify the claim that their work is their own.

I think that a constant thread can be found to run through all the examples I have given. For an analysand there is a great danger in establishing an object relation if he has idealized it, because it then assumes a magical omnipotence and the analysand gains the impression that he can never escape from it. Vertigo then intervenes, stopping the analysand from fulfilling his wish to establish this idealized object relationship, often by freezing it out, thus sparing him the dangers it entails. When this coveted relationship is less idealized and has lost its magical omnipotence, the analysand begins to consider the possibility of entering into it, and takes the more intense pleasure in it the more he feels that he can extricate himself from it again.

10

What makes a candidate for vertigo?

One might think that someone cured of vertigo would consider himself safe in a stable and solid world; he would, for instance, feel sure that he is not about to fall over, that the object will never drop him, that his relationship with his surroundings is so good that the world will never seem to totter about him or he to totter in it. Actually, the very opposite happens. I have noticed that being rid of vertigo, far from leading to a sense of tremendous stability, goes hand in hand with the de-idealization and acceptance of the vulnerability of the ego, of the object, and of their relationship.

What do we mean when we say someone has vertigo? Search for the specific characteristics of the symptom

While analysing Luc's vertigo, I followed the well-trodden path of the clinician: I started with his symptom and tried to understand its meaning and how he coped with it. But I also felt the need to follow another path, namely to discover why it is that, in grappling with similar circumstances and conflicts, some people get vertigo while others do not. I know quite well that the reasons underlying the choice of the symptom often perplex the analyst: once the symptom has appeared, he can often retrace the route by which it has arrived and help to make it go away again, but he may find it more difficult to see why, in apparently similar cases, the symptom fails to appear. In any case, I shall try to make clear what I believe to be specific about the symptom of vertigo of psychic origin.

*Asserting that vertigo is the price paid for immortalizing omnipotence
is not a specific enough explanation*

To set out as accurately as possible what characterizes the appearance of the symptom, I shall return to Luc's description of his first attack of vertigo and look at what he originally left out of his account.

It was towards the end of his analysis that Luc remembered what was apparently his first episode of vertigo. As a child, playing with his little friends, he had had no difficulty in clambering across a crossbar placed very high up in a very large room. As soon as he realized that he was higher up than everybody else, his present became all-pervasive – he knew nothing about the past any longer, nor about the future, about his climb or about how to get down again – he was on that crossbar for all eternity. The present froze Luc into eternal omnipotence. As soon as he had the grandiose feeling of being the biggest by some feat of magic, he unconsciously stopped time so as to remain the biggest for ever, but at that point he had an attack of vertigo. He had the impression that it was all a bit as if he had stopped a swing when it had carried him to its highest position: stopping its movement there meant he was bound to fall out. He also realized that when he overtook a car on the motorway, he froze time in much the same way and succumbed to vertigo. Luc then was the biggest for ever, but he was in danger of falling, of being castrated or of dying. Vertigo was the price he had had to pay for immortalizing a momentary and illusory feeling of omnipotence, but it was also an alarm signal putting him on his guard against the wish to be the biggest and the consequent threat of retaliation.

Now, many people grappling with their Oedipus complex experience moments of magical triumph like Luc, but not all of them have competition-related vertigo. Why is that? Is there something specific that causes vertigo to appear in one case and not in another?

A specific aspect of vertigo: omnipotent triumph dismissed as being derisory

Luc realized a little later that in his account of his crossbar experience he had left out a fleeting thought he had had up there on the crossbar: 'But in any case my brothers are bigger than me, they will always be the first-born.'

I then framed the hypothesis that it was at this point that Luc's attack of vertigo occurred; that is, during his inner confrontation with two voices he could not connect: a regressive voice and a more highly developed voice. Luc's regressive voice argued that his omnipotent infantile desire to overtake the whole world had been realized concretely because he was on top of the crossbar; that particular voice expressed an infantile aspect of himself which was content with the illusion that he was magically endowed with boundless omnipotence. The other voice reflected the reality principle; it expressed a more highly developed aspect of Luc, namely the realization that his brothers were bigger than he was and would, in any case, always be older; that voice reflected *a wish to wield realistic power* and involved the awareness of his relative smallness, and not his *wish to be omnipotent*. To this second voice, the triumph provided by magical omnipotence seemed derisory and could, in any case, provide no satisfaction.

Here we meet, on the psychic plane, the notion of incompatible data provided by different systems, the importance of which I stressed when discussing vertigo of somatic origin – one voice saying 'You are the biggest', and the other voice saying 'You are not the biggest'. For vertigo of psychic origin to appear, the simultaneous presence of two incompatible attitudes is essential: an infantile attitude of basking in illusory omnipotence and another more highly developed attitude that disdains such satisfaction.

In *An Outline of Psychoanalysis* (1940a [1938]), Freud points out that everyone can discover that he has two divergent attitudes. But I believe that *with the emergence of vertigo, an additional factor comes into play*: not only does the infantile part seek illusory fulfilment of its omnipotent wishes, but *this infantile part also bears witness to a very early fixation or regression, in which bodily expression prevails over verbalized expression*. This infantile part is based on early experiences of satisfaction of an omnipotent kind experienced through the body. Now, this additional factor helps to explain the somatic aspect of vertigo and the fact that this symptom recedes once representation and symbolization become possible.

I have noticed, in fact, that most of my analysands suffering from vertigo were able to report victories based on the feeling of magical omnipotence when they were babies; they seem to have felt these victories in their bodies: some of them even felt that they had been stronger than death, for instance because they had managed to be born while their brothers and sisters had died at birth before them, or again because they had managed to 'cling' to their mother's womb during her pregnancy and come into the world despite abortion attempts; others finally because they had survived potentially fatal diseases. Experiences of infantile omnipotence are very common, even though they are not always as extreme as those I have mentioned; this seems to accord with the frequency of the symptom of vertigo in the population at large.

I shall complete this hypothesis with the assumption that, while the infantile part seems to gain satisfaction, it may give the rest of the ego the impression that it is about to proliferate and hence to become invasive. I think that vertigo can, in that case, appear as an alarm signal preventing this infantile attitude from brimming over and swamping the whole personality. Vertigo may, in particular, allow the analysand to avoid a delusion of grandeur, that is mistaking illusory manifestations of omnipotence for manifestations of real power. In effect, we could see in Luc's case, that, if the infantile part assumes too great an importance and begins to invade, say, the sphere of professional activity, it poses a real threat. The longing for omnipotence, the quest for a magical realization at the professional level, can impede genuine professional success, which relies on trial and error rather than on magic.

This hypothesis explains why the transition from vertigo to equilibrium involves the de-idealization of the ego, of the object and of their relations; for the analysand, it means progressing from the register of infantile and magical omnipotence to that of realistic power. What I refer to as the *register of realistic power* corresponds to the attitude of an analysand who has the forward-looking desire to develop and deploy himself to the best of his ability and hence to be as powerful as possible within the confines of his own capacities; to that end he must bear the reality principle in mind, and in particular accept himself as he is, weaknesses and all.

To take this step, the analysand must reduce the discord between his two inner voices. On what basis can this reduction be effected? The relative importance the analysand attaches to his two inner attitudes may, for instance, change in favour of the progressive attitude and allow no more than a minimal influence to the regressive attitude, in such manner that the most highly developed side of the analysand will determine the object relationships by placing the various phantasies in an integrating context (for instance, fusion or triumph will no longer be experienced in the register of omnipotence but in a register reflecting reality and facilitating integrating activity); one could also imagine that the analysand's infantile part might develop in such a way that omnipotent satisfactions are no longer mistaken for concrete realizations, but become gradually accessible to symbolism, which entails a decrease in omnipotence and allows this infantile aspect to be brought into greater harmony with the rest of the ego. In any case, the prerequisite of a decrease in the inner discord is the recognition by the analysand that this infantile part belongs to him, and that it is only to the extent that it is correlated with the whole of his ego that it can develop. I believe that the two hypotheses I have framed are complementary.

In short, contrary to what one might think, there are two opposite cases in which vertigo does not arise: (1) when the infantile part is so omnipotent that no inner voice is raised against it; and (2) when the ego is sufficiently integrated for the infantile voice to be stripped of its despotic power. Vertigo appears in analysands who begin to see the illusory nature of omnipotent triumph, but have not yet renounced it strongly enough; in addition they must have gained the impression that their omnipotent wishes go back to an early physical experience of omnipotence.

The impossibility of linking omnipotence and realistic power

The search for illusory satisfaction at the level of magical omnipotence is made to the detriment of attempts to find satisfaction at the level of realistic power, because the latter means functioning to the best of one's real possibilities. Hence there is no way of linking the desire for omnipotence and the desire for real power. We can accept being a single, more or less unified, person, knowing that we shall always retain some more or less regressive or infantile aspects of an omnipotent kind, split or juxtaposed; we can hope to develop these parts or aspects or at least diminish their influence on the rest of the ego; but we shall find it impossible to link the affects springing from an infantile and regressive part of ourselves to those stemming from a developed part. They are not in the same register, are not part of the same argument.

When Luc believed that he was bigger than his brothers in his delusion of infantile omnipotence, yet realized that he was actually smaller than they were, these two views of reality could not be combined. He therefore had to renounce the illusory satisfaction before he could grow up. The reality principle stopped him from combining the pursuit of illusory satisfaction with the pursuit of realistic power. To discover the dynamism of growing up and becoming big like his daddy, the child must first realize that he is small. The analysand must similarly work over, and go beyond, his wishes for magical omnipotence, in order to adopt the register of his real possibilities.

I have been saying that every form of vertigo goes with a particular form of pleasure. Thus in fusion-related vertigo, the anxiety triggered by the idealized fusion goes with the pleasure of abandoning oneself to a brief spell of fusion. What precisely does the change from the one to the other involve?

In fact, the reason why I raise the relationship between a particular pleasure and the anxiety involved in a particular form of vertigo is that I realize that this relationship involves phenomena expressed on two distinct levels: in passing from vertigo to equilibrium we change register. The problem of vertigo is that, while the analysand's infantile part favours omnipotence, a more highly developed part of his ego favours realistic power. What he must do to get rid of his vertigo is not attempt to combine these two levels which are incompatible and mutually destructive, but on the contrary to ensure that his infantile part is allowed to mature or that its importance is relativized. For instance, as long as the analysand considers fusion in the register of omnipotence, he cannot combine it with any mode of object relationship, because in the first register fusion means either being swallowed up or the void, while in the second register it means that there is a relational space which is absent from the first. However, just as soon as the analysand considers fusion from a more mature standpoint and fusion no longer appears to be omnipotent, he can combine it with other modes of relationship and accord himself positive moments of fusion; this kind of pleasure must be placed in the context of an integrative attitude characteristic of the analysand's mature part. With it we abandon the register of vertigo for that of equilibrium; in fact, speaking of the search for equilibrium is perhaps just another way of speaking of the analysand's integrative ability. Actually, the concept of equilibrium is at the very heart of the perspective adopted by the most highly evolved part of the ego, and is characterized by the attempt to integrate opposites and to combine them. Thus, with an attitude based on realistic power, it is possible to combine, say, fusion and object relations, greatness and smallness, permanence and discontinuity. Omnipotence and realistic power, on the other hand, are not part of the same perspective and cannot be combined. It is in the analysand's more mature attitude that we first encounter the notion of equilibrium, thanks to which opposites can be combined into a synthetic creation.

What I have been saying in broad outlines for the sake of greater clarity must be amplified with the rich contributions provided by clinical encounters with analysands. Even if some of them, such as Luc, present clear splits between a regressive and a more or less highly developed part, many other analysands present a whole variety of attitudes or distinct aspects of the personality. For the rest, when I speak of a developed or mature part, I am fully aware that these things are relative, progressing or regressing, and that they vary according to the analysand's various interests.

It is thus that in the last chapter of this book, in which we shall be looking at the idea of equilibrium more closely, we shall find that when the ego, in its search for equilibrium, tries to combine opposites, it is constantly on the verge of leaning towards one or the other, thus ending up with disequilibrium every time. This is reminiscent of vertigo, but I shall refrain from calling it by that name and refer to it instead as a *sense of disequilibrium*, the better to account for the differences in the language in which vertigo and the sense of disequilibrium are expressed. Vertigo occurs in the presence of two elements that cannot be combined because they involve two distinct registers, while the sense of disequilibrium is produced in the presence of two elements that can be combined because they appear in one and the same register.

What does 'no longer having vertigo' mean on the clinical level?

De-idealization and renunciation of the ego's omnipotence leads to enhanced effectiveness

In the course of his analysis, an analysand's sense of identity develops to the extent that he succeeds in de-idealizing the notion of omnipotence. It may happen that a new analysand comes to analysis in the expectation that it will enable him not to make any more mistakes or to gain increasing magical power, and that, as a result, he will gain a greater sense of identity. Now, paradoxically, it is when the analysand abandons his magical need for omnipotence that he discovers that he is becoming more effective, because he then grasps that, within his own limits, he can exercise limited but certain power of his own. This recognition of his limits and of his vulnerability, far from being a sign that he is resigned to his smallness or has renounced his own worth, strengthens his sense of identity; it also improves his relationship with important objects because – the essential factor being that he becomes more and more himself in contact with them – the analysand has less need to idealize the objects with whom he used to identify himself or whom he used to copy.

How are we to understand the renunciation of omnipotence in connection with vertigo? We might, for example, imagine that a mountaineer who does not get vertigo at the top of a mountain must feel very sure of himself, and that he would start his descent into the valley without taking any unusual precautions, a little like the alpine choughs he sees flitting about in the sky around him. The mountaineer is not a chough, of course, but a human being, the kingdom of the air is not his to command. If he leapt down without any precautions, he would run the danger of injuring or even killing himself; this would be tantamount to a manic denial of the void and of his own limitations, not a sign of elaboration or integration of the data. His attitude would be almost comparable to that of a person paralysed by vertigo. By contrast, a mountaineer who is familiar with vertigo, and who has integrated his infantile magical wishes more fully, knows perfectly well that he is not a bird, tries to gauge his limitations, the difficulties of the descent, and takes every reasonable precaution to get down safely and soundly. We are reminded of Icarus who, by flying towards the sun with his wings made of wax and feathers, gave vain expression to his omnipotent and magical infantile wishes, while Daedalus, who respected his limitations and those of his mechanical inventions, was able to integrate them.

Renouncing the omnipotence of the object

An illusion: the reliable object must be infallible

We can observe to what large extent the analysand's idea of the reliability of the object develops hand in hand with a sense of his own identity. It often happens that, at the start of his analysis, the patient believes that he cannot rely on an object and consider it stable unless that object is infallible. He would, for example, love to have had parents who never made any mistakes, and believes that, in that case, he could really have trusted them and have introjected a stable object that would never have given him the impression that it might let him down; sometimes he even imagines that his parents' shortcomings are the sole cause of his inability to manage his life. He therefore idealizes the infallibility of the object and its omnipotence, and may have the illusion, at the beginning of his analysis, that the analyst is a repository of all truth. An omnipotent and infallible object may appear to be so immune to attacks that the analysand cannot imagine that the object might ever be affected by them, might ever disappear. He may even end up taking the object for granted, treating it as part of the decor and hence with the lack of respect reserved for solid pieces of furniture which, being in no imaginable danger, can 'take' whatever happens to them. Paradoxically once again, it is when the analysand discovers that the object is neither omnipotent nor infallible that he begins to appreciate its importance to him. The ephemeral character of the object and its vulnerability make him prize it all the more and treat it with greater care, continually surprised as he is at by its continued presence; he now looks as if he had discovered it for the first time.

A person aware of his fallibility can be trustworthy

In effect, the analysand discovers that the infallibility of the object is not synonymous with its trustworthiness, and that he can place his trust in an object that he knows perfectly well is capable of making mistakes. The fact that a person may err is therefore no longer an obstacle to his being trusted by the analysand; the important thing for the latter is, on the contrary, that that person should realize that he may be mistaken, and that he should manifestly be prepared to take this possibility into account. The de-idealization of the object does not mean that the analysand resigns himself to the smallness of the object but that he appreciates its value; this helps to open up to him horizons infinitely wider than illusory omnipotence can provide because it renders the object unique and hence irreplaceable. The analysand no longer needs blind faith in idealized objects: he dares to acknowledge that there are objects in which he has no trust; he allows himself to distinguish objects he considers trustworthy from those he does not, and he distinguishes between them not by virtue of their idealized infallibility or their omnipotence, but by the quality of the relations he believes he can establish with them.

The illusory belief in the omnipotence of the object is a corollary of the ego's wish for omnipotence

We saw that the mountaineer who has been able to integrate the feeling of vertigo remembers his own limitations; we shall see that he also remembers

134

the limitations of his equipment and of the people around him. He is not so reckless as to climb down a rock face putting blind trust in external objects. He checks the state of his abseiling rope and chooses his guide with care, knowing that guides are fallible people, and hence does his best to make sure he can rely on them and treat them as trustworthy objects. The way a mountaineer treats his external objects may be considered a reflection of his psychic world and of his inner attitude; in fact, his relations with outside objects somehow externalize the relations he has established with his internal objects – he has de-idealized them, and remembers their limitations.

All in all, the idealization of the object, the naive belief in its magical omnipotence, is often a corollary of the idealization of oneself. The analysand who wants to be omnipotent can project his ideal of omnipotence into the other, who is then turned into an ostensibly omnipotent object; this projective identification with an aggrandized object grants the analysand illusory fulfilment of his manic wishes.

11

Vertigo in the work of Sigmund Freud
and Melanie Klein

Sigmund Freud

Vertigo: 'An anxiety-equivalent'
(Freud 1916–1917: 401)

From his earliest writings, Freud has treated vertigo as a major manifestation of anxiety. In 1895, when he first described anxiety neurosis, he wrote: '"Vertigo" occupies a prominent place in the group of symptoms of anxiety neurosis. In its mildest form it is best described as "giddiness"; in its severer manifestations, as "attacks of vertigo" (with or without anxiety), it must be classed among the gravest symptoms of neurosis' (1895b: 95). Originally, Freud thought that this applied to locomotor vertigo only, but then he added: 'According to my observations, vertigo produced by heights, mountains and precipices is also often present in anxiety neurosis' (1895b: 96). Later Freud would often speak of the symptom of vertigo, either mentioning it on its own and assigning a specific symbolic meaning to it for a particular patient, or else placing it in the context of his general theory of anxiety. Thus he wrote in his *Introductory Lectures on Psychoanalysis*:

> The total [anxiety] attack can be represented by a single, intensely developed symptom, by a tremor, a *vertigo* [my italics; D.Q.], by palpitation of the heart, or by dyspnoea; and the general feeling by which we recognize anxiety may be absent or have become indistinct. Yet these conditions, which we describe as 'anxiety equivalents', have to be equated with anxiety in all clinical and aetiological respects.
>
> (1916–1917: 401)

Individual symbolic meanings of vertigo

To discover Freud's view on vertigo, we may feel tempted to present a pointillist canvas of his work and go in search of the individual symbolic meanings he attached to this symptom as presented by this or that patient of his. That approach may prove to be misleading: with it, we are in danger of looking for a *key to vertigo* much as so many people look for a *key to dreams*. We shall moreover discover quite quickly how much the meanings of vertigo can vary for Freud, and how wrong it would be to isolate just one and go on to infer Freud's opinion on vertigo in general from it. In fact, throughout his work, Freud makes brief references to particular forms of vertigo presented by some of his patients, and goes on to elucidate the symbolic meaning of this symptom. Though Freud invariably considers it a phobic manifestation of anxiety, we shall see that for him this manifestation assumed a different meaning with every patient, so that it would be idle to attach greater importance to one of these meanings than to any other.

I have chosen three examples to show that one and the same symptom of vertigo (fear of heights in the form of fear of windows) was interpreted by Freud in three quite distinct ways depending on the patient who presented it; in fact, during the interpretation, it is not the form of the symptom itself which matters most to him, but what each patient expresses by it. Here then are the three examples:

- *In 1896*, in his fifty-third letter to Fliess, Freud made his friend privy to his analysis of the 'fear of throwing oneself out of the window' present in one of his phobic patients: 'Unconscious idea: going to the window to beckon to a man as prostitutes do: sexual release arising from this idea. Preconsciousness: rejection, hence anxiety arising from the release of sexuality' (Freud 1887–1902: 181).
- *In 1922*, in 'Dreams and Telepathy', Freud likened this same symptom, that is the dread of an impulse to throw oneself out of a window, to the fear of heights, and argued that it was a fresh interpretation of childbirth (German: *Niederkunft* = coming down) (1922a: 213).
- *Then, in 1926*, in *Inhibitions, Symptoms and Anxiety*, Freud, referring to the same symptom, framed the hypothesis that drive anxiety may be a form of anxiety due not to the unused *libido* but to the unused *destructive drive*:

the instinctual demand before whose satisfaction the ego recoils is a masochistic one: the instinct of destruction directed against the subject himself. Perhaps an addition of this kind explains cases in which reactions of anxiety are exaggerated, inexpedient or paralysing. Phobias of heights (windows, towers, precipices and so on) may have some such origin. Their hidden feminine significance is closely connected with masochism.

(1926d: 168, addenda)

Freud's theories of anxiety

To discover what place vertigo occupies in Freud's work, it is much better to make a systematic study of his approach to the symptom than to look for particular references to it: since Freud treated vertigo as one of the most important manifestations of anxiety, we might try to determine what precise part vertigo plays in his general view of anxiety.

From 1893 to 1896, Freud did not think that anxiety, and hence vertigo, derived from any psychological source.

As early as 8 February 1893, in a letter to Fliess (1887–1902: 70) Freud mentions vertigo (giddiness on heights) as a chronic symptom of anxiety neurosis. But what does he have to say about anxiety itself?

At the time, Freud expressed the following idea which he maintained to the end of his life, namely that there is a connection between unused drive energy and the emergence of anxiety (letter of 17 November 1893, *ibid.*: 79); it should be added that the drive energy in question is the libido. However, in his earliest writings Freud insists on the purely *physical* and *direct* transformation of the unused libido into anxiety: 'Anxiety is to be connected not with a psychic but with a physical consequence of sexual abuse' (*ibid.*: 79–80). Freud supports this contention by pointing to patients who suffer frustration in their sexual life (for instance through coitus interruptus); he would explain later that at this period he believed that their neurotic anxiety arose out of unused libido and that it was thus 'related to it in the same kind of way as vinegar is to wine' (1905d: 224; note added in 1920), that is, by a completely non-psychic process.

Hence, at that time, Freud still believed that vertigo had non-psychic causes and did not, therefore, lend itself to treatment by psychoanalysis.

The pleasure of playing with vertigo (1900)

In *The Interpretation of Dreams* Freud deals with the question of vertigo in a highly original way. He refers to the pleasure of playing with vertigo, that is, of repeating *for fun*, in all tranquillity, a dangerous situation, the better to master it:

> There cannot be a single uncle who has not shown a child how to fly by rushing across the room with him in his outstretched arms, or who has not played by letting him fall . . . by holding him up high and then suddenly pretending to drop him. Children are delighted by such experiences and never tire of asking to have them repeated, especially when there is something about them that causes a little fright or giddiness.
>
> (1900a: 393)

Moreover, children are not alone in delighting in such experiences; to hear similar shouts of joy from adults, we have only to walk through a fairground. We may thus observe that, in children as well as in adults, the boundary between the pleasure provided by these games and the appearance of anxiety is very tenuous; mothers know well that sometimes these games end in tears, and that it takes very little for the cries of joy to make way quite suddenly for sobs.

Vertigo: a manifestation of phobic neurotic anxiety (1916–1917)

In his *Introductory Lectures on Psycho-Analysis* Freud tells us what place he assigns to vertigo among the various manifestations of anxiety. Moreover, it was at about the same time that he began to voice doubts about the validity of a purely physical theory of anxiety; in particular, he wrote that he could not understand how 'the anxiety which signifies a flight of the ego from its libido is after all supposed to be derived from that libido itself' (1916–1917: 405). The possibility of vertigo serving as part of a psychic defence mechanism thus began to be mooted.

In Lecture 25 of the same work, Freud gives a very detailed study of the various forms of anxiety, distinguishing in particular between realistic anxiety which 'corresponds to a reaction to danger' and 'neurotic anxiety in which danger plays little or no part' (*ibid.*: 401). To Freud, it is in the second category, that is, neurotic anxiety, that the symptom of vertigo must be placed; I shall accordingly take a closer look at this view.

Freud refers to a first form of neurotic anxiety as 'expectant anxiety'; it recurs in what he described as 'anxiety neurosis', and is characterized by 'a general apprehensiveness, a kind of freely floating anxiety, which is ready to attach itself to any idea that is in any way suitable' (*ibid.*: 398).

Freud contrasts this first type of neurotic anxiety with another type which he calls 'anxiety hysteria', to which he would also refer at times as phobic anxiety because it is characterized by phobias. This is a form of anxiety associated with certain objects or particular situations: the phobia replaces the internal threat, the dreaded libido, with an external danger. There is 'a projection outwards of the danger of libido' (*ibid.*: 410). It is to this phobic form of anxiety that Freud attaches the manifestations of vertigo.

What precise place does Freud assign to vertigo in phobic anxiety?

He distinguishes three types of phobia depending on the reality of the threat posed by the phobic object:

- Understandable phobias triggered off by a genuinely dangerous and sinister object or recalling a real danger, for instance snake phobia; in that case it is only the intensity of the reaction to the threat which seems exaggerated.

- Phobias 'in which the relationship to danger is still present, though we are accustomed to minimize the danger'; it is certain 'that we should fall into the river if the bridge collapsed at the moment we were crossing it; but that happens so exceedingly seldom that it does not arise as a danger' (*ibid.*: 399).
- The third group of phobias 'is quite beyond our comprehension. When a strong, grown-up man is unable owing to anxiety to walk along a street or cross a square in his own familiar home-town . . . how are we to relate these things to the danger which they obviously constitute for the phobic subject?' (*ibid.*: 399–400). In this connection, Freud mentions agoraphobia, which often goes hand in hand with vertigo. It is, in any case, a symptom, a fear of empty space, which prevents the patient from taking a walk that might entail an imaginary danger.

The reason why Freud called phobic neurosis *anxiety hysteria*, at the risk of confusing it with conversion hysteria, was to draw attention to the constituent elements of that neurosis, and to underline its structural similarity to conversion hysteria. In Freud's own words: 'We class all these phobias as *anxiety hysteria*; that is to say, we regard them as a disorder closely related to the familiar conversion hysteria' (*ibid.*: 400). However, though they are similar, they nevertheless remain distinct, and the reason why I stress this fact is that I realize how difficult it may be, during the first contact with a patient suffering from vertigo of psychic origin, to distinguish between phobic manifestations and hysterical (conversion) manifestations; colleagues faced with the physical character of the vertigo crisis may sometimes gain an early impression that they might be dealing with a case of hysteria. Freud himself set the example: at the beginning of his career, before having studied anxiety neurosis, he thought that the attacks of giddiness of one of his first patients might be hysterical (1895d: 112–13). Later, when he had studied phobias, he no longer hesitated in placing these attacks, and vertigo in general, among the manifestations of phobic anxiety.

On the subject of the difference between anxiety hysteria (phobia) and conversion hysteria, *The Language of Psycho-Analysis* has this to say:

> The job of repression in both cases is essentially to separate affects from ideas. There is nevertheless an essential difference between the two conditions, which Freud emphasizes: in anxiety hysteria, the libido which has been liberated from the pathogenic material by repression is not *converted* . . . but is set free in the shape of anxiety.
>
> (Laplanche and Pontalis 1973: 38)

This distinction is clinically justified: the analysand who has an attack of vertigo suffers from anxiety.

Moreover, in 1916, Freud already spoke of object loss as the precondition

of the appearance of anxiety; he likened the anxiety of the adult to that of
the child

who is frightened of a strange face because he is adjusted to the sight of
a familiar and beloved figure – ultimately of his mother. It is his disappointment and longing that are transformed into anxiety – his libido,
in fact, which has become unemployable, which cannot at that time be
held in suspense and is discharged as anxiety.

(1916–1917: 407)

Vertigo has a psychic component; the ego is the actual seat of anxiety (1926d)

From his *Inhibitions, Symptoms and Anxiety* (1926d) onwards, Freud considered that 'the ego is the actual seat of anxiety' (1926d: 140). This topical
definition is very important, because it restores the idea that a psychic act is
involved in the formation of anxiety, and hence of vertigo. Freud thus
renounced his earlier view that 'anxiety arises directly out of libido' (*ibid.*:
141). In fact, whereas 'at one time I attached some importance to the view
that what was used as a discharge of anxiety was the cathexis which had
been withdrawn in the process of repression', Freud's new view was that
'anxiety is an affective state and as such can, of course, only be felt by the
ego' (*ibid.: 140*). This new conception is very important in the analysis of
vertigo; vertigo, being equivalent to phobic neurotic anxiety, now had a psychic component and was therefore susceptible to psychoanalysis.

According to Freud, 'anxiety is a signal given by the ego in order to affect
the pleasure–unpleasure agency' (*ibid.*: 140) when it senses danger or the
threat of danger. In accordance with this new theory, the condition determining anxiety can be likened to the threat of the loss of a loved object
(*ibid.*: 81). This object loss has different meanings according to the level of
libidinal development to which the patient assigns it. For example, in the
case of castration anxiety, it is the upsurge of genital libido that is feared,
whereas in the case of the infant's fear of solitude a less highly developed
instinctual force is involved. Freud put it even more clearly in the *New
Introductory Lectures on Psycho-Analysis* (1933a). This is very important for the
understanding of the diversity of the symbolic meanings of the symptom of
vertigo, which corresponds to the diversity of the dangers, themselves corresponding to the various meanings assumed by object loss and also to the
various drives involved.

Freud points out for the first time that, during the appearance of anxiety,
the drive before which the ego recoils, and which therefore remains unemployed, is not necessarily the libido, but may also be 'the instinct of destruction

directed against the subject himself' (1926d: 168, note 1); I would recall that he mentions that phobias of height may be of similar origin.

Psychic origin of anxiety and hence of vertigo (1933a)

The vertigo alarm signal

In his *New Introductory Lectures on Psycho-Analysis* (1933a) Freud devotes Lecture 32 to the recapitulation, modification and completion of what he had written in the *Introductory Lectures on Psycho-Analysis* of 1916–1917. He reintroduces the idea that neurotic anxiety springs from the direct transformation of libido into anxiety (1933a: 83), but uses a new perspective: what is involved is no longer a direct physical transformation, but a transformation effected by the ego and involving mental energy. In fact, Freud now takes account of the fact that the psychic personality is made up of a superego, an ego and an id, which correspond to three types of anxiety (real, neurotic and moral), which, in turn,

> can be so easily connected with the ego's three dependent relations – to the external world, to the id and to the super-ego. Along with this new view, moreover, the function of anxiety as a signal announcing a situation of danger . . . comes into prominence.
>
> (*ibid.*: 85)

Freud has come to consider it an important point that the transformation of libido into anxiety should be of psychic origin. Anxiety is a defence mechanism, put into operation by the ego as an alarm signal against such external dangers as loss of the object, loss of love, or the threat of castration; the question of what anxiety is made up of has lost its interest; now these threats coming from the outside are themselves elicited by the internal threat constituted by the drive (itself perhaps rendered all the more disturbing if, being deprived of its object of satisfaction, it remains unemployed). This situation created by the drive has now become a prime threat, this time from within. Ultimately, what a person is afraid of (in neurotic anxiety) 'is evidently his own libido' (*ibid.*: 84).

Does every age of development involve a different type of vertigo?

Freud shows that every age of development goes with a given state of anxiety, from which we may take it that every age of development goes with a specific form of vertigo.

What makes this view of anxiety so interesting is that it brings out the diversity of the forms of anxiety and of the threats against which the ego defends itself according to the level of development of the drives involved; moreover we rediscover this diversity in our study of the equivalent of anxiety, namely vertigo. But let us see how Freud himself puts it:

> we can say that in fact a particular determinant of anxiety (that is, situation of danger) is allotted to every age of development as being appropriate to it. The danger of psychical helplessness fits the stage of the ego's early immaturity; the danger of loss of an object (or loss of love) fits the lack of self-sufficiency in the first years of childhood; the danger of being castrated fits the phallic phase; and finally fear of the super-ego, which assumes a special position, fits the period of latency. In the course of development the old determinants of anxiety should be dropped, since the situations of danger corresponding to them have lost their importance owing to the strengthening of the ego. But this only occurs most incompletely . . . There is no doubt that the people we describe as neurotics remain infantile in their attitude to danger and have not surmounted obsolete determinants of anxiety.
>
> (*ibid.*: 88–89)

The above quotation is reminiscent of something Freud wrote seven years earlier in *Inhibitions, Symptoms and Anxiety* (1926d: 138). But a closer reading brings out an interesting difference: in 1926d the infant's fear of loneliness (which can persist in adult neurotics) is still an automatic, purely physical, anxiety for Freud, whereas in 1933a he explains that 'this infantile anxiety must . . . be regarded not as of the realistic but as of the neurotic kind' (1933a: 83). We can therefore see that Freud came to attach increasingly great importance to the role of the psyche, from which it follows that even the most regressive manifestation of the symptom of vertigo can be considered susceptible to psychoanalysis.

It should be noted that Freud, in 1933a, was concerned with distinguishing the anxiety from the symptom that may accompany it: 'It seems, indeed, that the generation of anxiety is the earlier and the formation of symptoms the later of the two, as though the symptoms are created in order to avoid the outbreak of the anxiety state' (1933a: 84). This comment is particularly relevant to our study of vertigo. In fact, in Freud's view the symptom of vertigo represents the attempt to avoid the sudden eruption of the state of anxiety, since in principle all the analysand need do to protect himself against it is to avoid places likely to give him vertigo.

Vertigo as a manifestation of various forms of anxiety; the importance of splitting in the emergence of vertigo (1940a [1938])

In *An Outline of Psycho-Analysis* (1940a [1938]), Freud sums up the essential views on anxiety at which he arrived towards the end of his life. He repeats, in particular, that 'it [the ego] makes use of the sensations of anxiety as a signal to give a warning', and explains that this warning is against 'dangers that threaten its integrity' (*ibid.*: 199).

Above all, however, Freud sets out at the end of this work the idea of the *splitting of the ego* which I mentioned in Chapter 1 and in several clinical examples as being of great importance in the study of vertigo. The idea of the splitting of the ego lies at the very heart of what constitutes the specific character of vertigo, since vertigo ensues, according to my observations, when two attitudes are present simultaneously in the ego: an infantile attitude seeking satisfaction in the register of omnipotence, and a more highly developed attitude seeking satisfaction in the register of potency, a register in which the triumph of the first attitude is considered to be derisory.

Were Freud's blackouts instances of vertigo?

In September 1912, Freud complained in letters to Binswanger and Jones of heart complaints following smoking and the drinking he had added to it while on holiday. 'And so I suppose the heart rebelled; everyone will now construe psychic influence to account for this' (quoted by Schur 1972: 265).

However, in Munich, on 24 November 1912, it was no longer a case of a general indisposition: Freud had a fainting spell during a meal with Jung, Jones, Abraham and some other colleagues. He first referred to it as an 'anxiety crisis', so much so that he stressed the anxiety rather than the fainting spell it was supposed to have caused. This episode led him to wonder about other illnesses he had previously had and which he had formerly attributed mainly to somatic causes. 'I had an anxiety attack at the table, similar to the one I had had at the Essighaus [restaurant] in Bremen. I tried to get up and fainted for a moment' (letter to Ferenczi, quoted in *ibid.*: 266). A few days later, he wondered about the immediate causes and the psychic background. He wrote to Jones on 8 December 1912:

> I cannot forget that six and four years ago I suffered from a very similar though not as intense symptom in the *same* room of the Park Hotel. I saw Munich first when I visited Fliess during his illness and this town seems to have acquired a strong connection with my relation to that man. There is some piece of unruly homosexual feeling at the root of the matter.
>
> (*ibid.*: 267)

Freud mentioned this episode on two subsequent occasions but no longer referred to it as either a fainting fit or an anxiety crisis, but as giddiness or attacks of *vertigo*. He attached increasing attention to the psychic motives and referred to the somatic conditions of the symptom as 're-enforcing' causes. Thus he wrote to Ferenczi on 9 December 1912: 'I have fully regained my capacity to work, have analytically settled the dizzy spell [vertigo] in Munich . . . All these attacks point to the significance of very early experiences with death (in my case a brother who died very young, when I was a little over one year old)' (*ibid.*: 267–8). On 1 January 1913, he wrote to Binswanger:

My fainting attack [vertigo] in Munich was surely provoked by psychogenic elements, which received strong somatic re-enforcements (a week of troubles, a sleepless night, the equivalent of a migraine, the day's tasks) . . . Repressed feelings, this time directed against Jung, as previously against a predecessor of his, naturally play the main part.

(*ibid.*: 268)

Freud was to mention another attack of severe dizziness he suffered on his seventy-seventh birthday. He wrote to Marie Bonaparte: 'Dr. Schur, who by chance came in right afterwards, did not make much of it. His diagnosis asserted that the dizziness was of a vestibular type and caused by nicotine' (letter of 9 May 1933, *ibid.*: 445). However, it seems clear that, for Freud, the feelings aroused by his birthday played a part in the occurrence of these episodes because, a year later, he wrote to Marie Bonaparte that when he thought of the dizziness during his last birthday, he dreaded the approach of the next one (letter of 2 May 1934).

Max Schur, Freud's disciple, friend and personal physician, mentions a hypothesis by Jones which fits in with my own observations: to Jones these attack of giddiness were the tribute Freud had to pay for an illusory victory. Jones, in fact, had revealed that in Bremen as well as in Munich, Freud had fainting spells after a small victory over Jung: in Bremen, Freud had been able to persuade Jung to give up his strict teetotalism, whereupon Jung had assured him of his loyalty; in Munich, Freud had criticized Jung very strongly, and Jung had apologized. This enabled Schur to write: 'Jones interpreted the occurrence of both fainting spells after the achievement of a small victory as evidence that Freud was paying a price for that victory. Similarly he viewed Freud's own analysis of the episode which pointed to the death of his brother Julius, as paying for "the success of defeating an opponent"' (*ibid.*: 270).

We might add that the inconvenience of vertigo also helps to stop those afflicted with it from succumbing to an omnipotent drive for glory that threatens to rebound on them in the form of dire punishment. But I would add above all, with respect to my hypothesis about the specific nature of vertigo, that such victories may have appeared as such to only a regressive part of Freud's ego, and that to the rest of his personality they looked more like infantile victories on the omnipotent level. Jones, moreover, spoke of 'small victories'. In effect, Freud doubtless had no need to bolster his fame with a victory consisting, for example, in persuading Jung to take a little wine with his meals. I accordingly frame the hypothesis that his vertigo appeared when Freud discovered the derisory character of the omnipotent feeling his regressive part obtained from these petty triumphs. This brings me back to my hypothesis that vertigo appears when two tendencies coexist, a regressive part of the ego turning a simple small victory into illusory omnipotence, while the rest of the ego, which relies on potency and not on omnipotence, takes stock of the infantile character of the idealization of this small triumph. I would therefore frame the further hypothesis that vertigo might intervene to stop this illusion of omnipotence from assuming too much importance.

The search for the meaning, by Freud and his followers, of what he called his dizzy spells is interesting for a variety of reasons. In fact, it is not simply when he speaks in theoretical vein that Freud considers vertigo as a manifestation of anxiety; he does the same when describing concrete personal experiences since, in accounting for his fainting episodes, he refers to them as anxiety crises as well as vertigo crises. I might also mention that the more time Freud devoted to the analysis of what had happened to him, the more he seemed to consider fainting or giddy spells as the somatic aspect of a psychic state. Moreover, though Freud attached such importance to the search for the psychic significance of this manifestation of anxiety, he nevertheless recalled its bodily basis. We thus rediscover at the level of personal experience what Freud affirmed in theory and what I have quoted on several occasions: 'The ego is first and foremost a bodily ego'.

Melanie Klein: theoretical concepts supporting my own view of vertigo

Vertigo being a manifestation of anxiety, as we have seen, the contribution by Melanie Klein to the psychoanalytic theory of anxiety has helped me a great deal in my attempts to interpret the various aspects of that symptom. That is why, even though she did not refer to vertigo directly – perhaps because, unlike Freud she did not suffer from it except briefly at the end of her life – I shall single out those points of her theory that have helped to support my own study.

The longing for lost unity

People suffering from fusion-related vertigo idealize fusion, often considered as the return to the primitive unity with one's mother. Now, Melanie Klein postulates a universal longing for the sense of security accompanying the pre-natal state: 'It may well be that his having formed part of the mother in the pre-natal state, contributes to the infant's innate feeling that there exists outside him something that will give him all he needs and desires' (1957: 3). But this desire for idealized fusion can only lead to frustration. In effect, for Melanie Klein, persecutory anxiety is stirred up by birth and may possibly extend to the unborn infant's unpleasant experiences in the womb (*ibid.*: 4). Moreover, even if the infant's longing for an omnipresent breast were satisfied, it would only lead to frustration and anxiety: the infant needs to lose and to regain the good object to discover his love for it. This shows that the *experiences of being dropped* and of *ego–object differentiation* are needed if the infant is to appreciate that equilibrium must constantly be restored.

For Melanie Klein frustration is indispensable if we are to experience the innate conflict between love and hate, which culminates in the conflict between the life and death drives. I believe firmly that when patients love life, it is not because they are basking in good fortune, but because they have acquired a taste for the struggle involved in becoming oneself through relations with important whole objects. Thus one analysand negotiated every difficulty in her life as if it were an obstructive passage she had to negotiate before she could start to live at long last; but after every problem solved she invariably imagined another, and she always expected to start living 'afterwards'. When would that be? When there were no more problems left to solve? On her death? And she wondered if that was all there was to life, this struggle to live in the present. These ideas are important to bear in mind if we are to appreciate that it is in opposition to change that vertigo intervenes, while movement encourages a sense of stability.

Two forms of anxiety that may cause different types of vertigo

Melanie Klein distinguishes between two forms of anxiety, namely persecutory anxiety characteristic of the paranoid-schizoid position and depressive anxiety characteristic of the depressive position. For her these two forms of anxiety and these two positions are the expression of the duality of drives present from the beginning of life: destructive drives and organizing drives, splitting and integrating drives, death and life drives. What interests me above all is to discover how different analysands try to fit this duality of drives into their history and are able to express it through the particular form they give to, for example, a particular symptom of vertigo.

Persecutory anxiety is rooted in the fear of annihilation of the ego (Klein 1948). The splitting of the object into an idealized object and a devalued object, which is characteristic of this type of anxiety, occurs above all in fusion-related vertigo, vertigo related to being dropped, suction-related vertigo and expansion-related vertigo. In fact, these forms of vertigo do not (or hardly ever) involve a relational space: the idealized object can suddenly turn into a devalued object that becomes annihilated, drops, sucks in or collides. Clinical practice thus brings us into contact with analysands who suffer because they suddenly change from trust in an idealized environment to deep despair about what feels like a hostile environment. This *swing*, often triggered off by the slightest intervention, leaves these patients in a state of disarray, sometimes expressed through the insupportable vertiginous feeling. The need to idealize the object reflects the ego's need to love itself in idealized form only. The analysand is torn between love of his idealized self and rejection of his devalued self; this can entail a process of flight and attraction as in *vertigo related to imprisonment and escape*, or create the conditions needed for the appearance of *vertigo related to attraction to the void*: the analysand has emptied himself of what he does not love in himself and has cast it out.

Melanie Klein shows that the disadvantages of the splitting associated with the paranoid-schizoid position give rise to the re-enforcement of the other tendency of the ego which, by contrast, aims at the integration and linkage of the split parts. It is then that *depressive anxiety* emerges which 'is related above all to the damage inflicted on the loved internal and external objects by the subject's destructive impulses' (1948). Hence, if the *persecutory anxiety* about the destruction of the ego diminishes, the *depressive anxiety* about harming or losing the object increases. The change from a feeling of emptiness to a feeling of space reflects the characteristic fear of damaging the good object associated with depressive anxiety. Not only the analytic atmosphere changes but also the quality of the analysand's life – instead of being constantly on the defensive, the patient starts to take an interest in the people around him. We shall rediscover this process when we come to look at the constitution of psychic space in vertigo related to attraction to the void.

Elaboration of the depressive position

The fresh upsurge of depressive anxiety when persecutory anxiety diminishes may convey the impression that the ego has fallen between Scylla and Charybdis. Must the ego necessarily regress into *confusion*, muddling up affects and proving incapable of deciding whether it loves or detests this indistinct global object, in order to alleviate the disadvantages of persecutory anxiety while avoiding depressive anxiety? Such regression would entail a third danger, namely a state of mental disorder.

This inability to extricate oneself from between persecutory anxiety and depressive anxiety encourages the emergence of vertigo related to imprisonment–escape and above all competition-related vertigo. In fact, as I mentioned in Chapter 8, I have often seen vertigo appear the moment an analysand realized that he no longer felt love *or* hatred for a unique object, but love *and* hatred; this combination seemed impossible to him. His feelings involved a unique object, but one whose apparently 'total' character was due to a juxtaposition of its various aspects, and not to their synthesis, which would have created an object with a different qualitative character. He could only split or juxtapose his love and hatred, having failed to consider the possibility of associating them and thus creating a new feeling with a quality distinct from that of its two components. I have always felt that this moment in the not yet worked-through depressive position lends itself to episodes of vertigo; it is a delicate, or even dangerous, moment, because the analysand may be tempted to act out (D. Quinodoz 1984a), especially by means of accidents that I have sometimes considered the equivalents of vertigo.

To avoid this triple danger and to work through the depressive position, the analysand must discover what the love-synthesis directed at the total object perceived as a *whole* person means to him. That discovery opens the analysand up to a relationship of a *new quality* with his internal objects, and to a reorganization of his sense of equilibrium.

The moment of integration can be described, but is difficult to explain

This moment of integration, when the analysand abandons an object relationship based on a *love balance sheet* (which involves adding up the good sides of the object and then deducting the sum of the bad sides, so as to weigh up if the object is lovable) for a relationship based on a *love-synthesis*, seems to me to have the character of a psychic creation. The intangible aspect of the integration takes one back to what is intangible in the insight of patients who discover the meaning of their vertigo. Thus Luc's reaction upon discovering that his centre of gravity did not lie outside but inside him, might well have been anticipated, but the discovery itself had the character of a creative act and not of something rationally explicable. His response was in fact reminiscent of the way we respond to a melody: we hear a juxtaposition of notes, but sometimes the miracle occurs, and we find ourselves listening to a melody.

I believe that an analysand can have this integrative experience in his contacts with the analyst when he feels, during analytic sessions, that every element of the material he produces recalls the whole of his person to the analyst, and that every element, when it makes full sense, is placed by the analyst into a whole that cannot be mistaken for any other. This strikes me as being comparable to the experience of music lovers: they would never mistake one of Sydney Bechet's phrases for a passage from a Beethoven symphony. I think that when a person dares to enter upon the long adventure of a psychoanalysis, he does so, among other reasons, because he has seen the possibility of discovering in it, in contact with the analyst, an original and irreplaceable dimension that turns him into a unique person with a worth greatly superior to what he believed could be rationally expected.

Stability and equilibrium for Melanie Klein

Melanie Klein has stressed that 'externalization of internal danger situations is one of the ego's earliest methods of defence against anxiety and remains fundamental in development' (1948). Now, the vertigo experienced before the external void may well be a defence against the anxiety triggered off by the internal void.

Melanie Klein has, moreover, given a striking description of this mechanism when discussing the case of the painter Ruth Kjär who, when suddenly plunged into the deepest melancholy, said: 'There is an empty space in me which I can never fill!' (1929: 215). This woman managed to externalize her inner void the day someone had taken away a picture she loved, leaving 'an empty space on the wall, which in some inexplicable way seemed to coincide with the empty space within her' (*ibid.*: 215). She was then able to examine the empty space which, while it had remained purely internal, had filled her with too much anxiety to face: 'The empty space grinned hideously down at her' (*ibid.*: 215). Now she could set about repairing this internal object she had externalized. She began to put paint on the empty space on the wall, thus restoring life to what she had imagined had been annihilated inside her: the mother she believed she had destroyed as well as the part of herself destroyed by her mother.

Though Melanie Klein did not use the term 'vertigo' as such, she examined the sense of stability and equilibrium, two complements of vertigo. She describes, for example, the failure of schizophrenics to ensure their own stability.

> The schizophrenic feels that he is hopelessly in bits and that he will never be in possession of his self. The very fact that he is so fragmented results in his being unable to internalize his primal object (the mother) sufficiently as a good object and therefore in his lacking the foundation of stability; he cannot rely on an internal and external good object nor can he rely on his own self.
>
> (1963: 103–4)

I believe that, from the most primitive forms of vertigo on, the analysand experiences, in a split-off part of his ego, the breakdown of the process ensuring his own stability, while this process can develop quite normally in the remainder of his ego. The process itself has been described very clearly by Hanna Segal:

> At every step the battle must be waged anew between, on the one hand, regression from the depressive pain to the paranoid-schizoid mode of functioning or, on the other, a working through of the depressive pain leading to further growth and development . . . But the degree to which the depression has been worked through and internal good objects securely established within the ego determines the maturity and stability of the individual.
>
> (1979: 135–6)

'The central task of the infant's elaboration of the depressive position is to establish in the core of his ego a sufficiently good and secure whole internal object' (*ibid.*: 80).

12

Dangerous games with vertigo

Risking a fall or dicing with death? Players of impossible games

Different games

There are several ways of playing with vertigo: sometimes the risk is minimal, at worst a bad fall, for instance from a fairground roundabout, or while waltzing, or mountaineering with a stout rope. By contrast, skiing down a near-vertical slope, or walking a tightrope between the Trocadero and the Eiffel Tower, means running considerable risks as the slightest mistake may prove fatal.

One can also play different games with vertigo in other fields. For example, some patients get thrills without taking serious risks in their business affairs or financial operations: all they risk is surplus they can easily spare. Others risk everything. Like skiers who go down near-vertical slopes, they might be called financiers of the impossible. A great variety of risks can also be run in the artistic field, even though not quite so patently. I have seen this happen with some of my patients, but not in its most acute form, because I have never had 'artists of the impossible' as analysands. However, I have been intrigued by the accounts of some of my painter friends and also by the questions raised by the suicides of such artists as Vincent van Gogh and Nicolas de Staël.

Vincent van Gogh

The swirling olive trees, cypresses, wheat fields, stars or suns that blaze out from some of van Gogh's canvases have often given me the impression that van Gogh's inner world was in constant turmoil as he went in search of the unattainable balance that would have allowed him to find his true place. The conditions in which van Gogh started his life made it hard for him to gain a sense of his own identity: he was called Vincent like the brother who had been born a year to the day before him and who had died at birth; he was assigned his dead brother's number in the local register of births and deaths and, at a very early age, he was able to read that the grave, beside the little church in which his father officiated, was that of Vincent van Gogh . . . Who was the real Vincent van Gogh? Which one was alive? Could the one take the place of the other?

The point I am trying to make is this: what we can see in the canvases van Gogh painted during his great and last crisis, shortly before his suicide, seems to illustrate the metaphor used by Luc to express the role of psychic immobilization in his attacks of vertigo: while the swing is in motion those sitting on it run no danger, but if it is suddenly stopped at the highest point it can reach, they are easily thrown out. In fact, van Gogh's last great crisis coincided with the birth of his nephew Vincent: one might have expected that the artist's unstable world would reel even more at the arrival of a new Vincent van Gogh, his brother Theo's son. Thus around 20 February 1890, the artist wrote to his mother: 'I should have much preferred if he had named his son after Pa . . . than after me' (1990: 2023). Even so, it was not a reeling scene that van Gogh captured on his canvas; instead, he presented his nephew with *Blossoming Almond Tree*, a work that seemed to radiate balance and peace under an unclouded blue sky. The inner turmoil had apparently abated, but I think that the appearances were misleading: van Gogh had merely stopped the swing – perhaps, in order to keep up his welcoming uncle front, he halted the movement of the drive, froze it but without being able to integrate it, and barely had he finished that painting than he was brought low. As soon as he had recovered some of his lucidity, he tried to tell his brother something about that painting: 'You will see that the last canvas with the branches in blossom was perhaps the best, the one on which I worked most patiently, painted calmly and with a greater assurance of touch. And the next day I was completely done in' (letter of April 1890; van Gogh 1996: 483).

Van Gogh killed himself three months later. I think that creating a visual representation of his dizzy inner world might have helped him to keep his swing in balance a bit longer. But once it stopped moving, he was brought face to face with death.

Nicolas de Staël

Nicolas de Staël's case seems to be quite different. His premature death was undoubtedly related to the problem he had in fitting his past into his present in order to build his own internal history. The fact that he burned almost everything he had painted before 1942 could therefore be considered a reflection of a more general attitude, of an unconscious scorched earth policy, as if in suppressing his sad past, he hoped to protect his present; but in so doing he rendered his work of mourning exceedingly difficult.

In any case, what I wish to stress here is more directly connected with vertigo. Nicolas de Staël killed himself by jumping out of a window; he flung himself physically into that space he had so often tried to plumb in his work, by presenting it sometimes as flat, without any perspective, and sometimes possessed of an infinite, immaterial depth. Difficult though I find it, not being an artist, to understand how a painter is able to relive vertigo in a vital or mortal manner in his painting, I can imagine that painters, and no doubt other artists as well, can play with vertigo in their work to the point of dicing with death. That is why I was shattered to read what de Staël wrote to Jacques Dubourg towards the end of December 1954, three months before his suicide: 'What I am trying for is continuous renewal, truly continuous and that is not easy. I know what my painting is beneath its appearances, its violence, its perpetual play of forces, namely a fragile thing in the good, the sublime sense. It is fragile like love, I believe inasmuch as I can control myself, I always try to turn my possibilities as a painter more or less into decisive action and when I throw myself into a large canvas, if it turns out well, I always feel atrociously too large a role on the part of chance, like a vertigo, a chance in the force that preserves despite everything, its face of chance, its reverse side of virtuosity, and that always puts me into lamentable states of discouragement. I do not manage to persevere, and even the three-metre canvases on which I place a few strokes a day, thinking about it, always end up in vertigo . . . If the vertigo, to which I cling as to an attribute of quality, were to shift gently towards greater precision, more freedom, out of harassment, one would have a brighter day' (1981). A few weeks later, de Staël jumped to his death. Between which pleasure and what anxiety did his vertigo veer?

Marcelle Spira has told me (personal communication) that what struck her most about Nicolas de Staël was his ability to express transparency, and that she wondered if that might not have been the painter's way of projecting an inner feeling of being transparent himself. That led me to try and puzzle out what precisely the artist meant by vertigo in his letter to Jacques Dubourg. Was he not trying to project onto canvas his feeling of being a luminous transparency traversing all objects and thus expanding endlessly in a world without end? But did he not also project his opposite desire of being stopped by solid, concrete, heavy objects? When he wrote to Dubourg, 'I am trying to capture still lifes . . .', was he not trying, through his painting of these objects, to feel in himself the solidity of his own existence (November 1954)? Was he not trying to effect a difficult synthesis between his wish to expand immaterially in a world without end and the wish to drop to the ground like a ponderous object? I have the impression that this longing for synthesis ended up in a distressing juxtaposition found in one of his last paintings: *Railway Beside the Sea at Sunset*. Standing before this fine work in which the massive black train hurtles against the immaterial light of the setting sun and the sea stretching to infinity, I can sense the vertiginous clash of the irreconcilable.

On 18 December 1954, a few weeks before his suicide, de Staël wrote to Dubourg: 'When I shall have finished the transparencies, I shall go on to the beetroots, and I may or may not keep the matching ground to the end.' De Staël's dramatic experiences with vertigo at the time were perhaps connected with the third form of ambivalence which I have called transitory; de Staël tried to paint either transparent effects (his feeling of immaterial lightness) or the beetroots (his feeling of concrete weight), but he did not think it possible to combine them. I believe that the feeling of transparent immateriality without the sense of weight might have weakened his sense of identity and have given him the impression that he himself lacked gravity.

Had he been able to externalize on canvas his need to experience the synthesis of his longing for lightness and his longing for weight, that is, had he managed to paint vertigo 'with more freedom, out of harassment', he might perhaps have spared himself the leap into space that cost him his life – perhaps in an attempt to take wing even while pressing down on the ground? Just before his death, he wrote to Dubourg: 'I am unique only thanks to that leap which I have just put to canvas with more or less contact' (17 February 1955). Might his last leap have missed the canvas?

The challenge to death does not always lie where one thinks it does

Analysands who like braving fate and take great pleasure in playing dangerous games with vertigo often make one wonder whether they like having brushes with death. What link is there between that attitude and the death drive? Some patients take pleasure in brushes with death like drug addicts, or in pain like masochists, but that does not seem to be the essential point. I shall make every effort not to simplify the situation and not to see those flirting with death in places where they do not happen to be.

The duality of drives: life drive and death drive

Freud has postulated the presence of an original, fundamental conflict, involving the most primitive forms of psychic activity, expressed by the confrontation of the life drive, the constructive force favouring the creation and maintenance of ever greater unities, and the death drive which encourages the destruction of vital unities and the return to the inorganic state. Now, it is the problem of the creation and destruction of vital unities by the life and death drives respectively which impinges most closely on our patients' possible challenge to death: do they manage to associate these two drives or do they keep them apart? Here we come up against several ambiguities.

Generally, it is perfectly clear that the separation of the life and death drives entails a degree of destructiveness: while the combination of the life and death drives serves vital processes, their separation has the opposite effect. 'In biological functions the two basic instincts operate against each other or combine with each other. Thus, the act of eating is a destruction of the object with the final aim of incorporating it, and the sexual act is an act of aggression with the purpose of the most intimate union' (Freud 1940a [1938]: 149).

We have everyday examples of this need to combine the life and death drives for the preservation of vital processes: it is essential to our survival that some of our cells should keep dying while others keep being born; the surgeon who performs an appendectomy also combines the destructive drive (opening the abdomen) with the love drive (pain relief) in his attempt to save life; that operation could not dispense with either drive; by contrast, the gangster who slashes the belly of his victim does so with a destructive drive not bound up with Eros, and the result does not benefit vital processes.

However, in some cases we might gain the impression that the association of the life and death drives entails a degree of destructiveness. Thus we could say that there is a link between the death drive and the sexual impulse in masochism, or in drug addiction because, in these cases, there is an eroticization of the death drive leading to sexual pleasure in causing pain or death; the drug addict thinks of his lethal drug as a delight, a paradise; he enjoys taking it, much as the masochist enjoys pain. Masochism and drug addiction are essentially destructive.

Two ways of combining the two drives

What are we to think? Is destructiveness – auto-destructiveness or hetero-destructiveness – due to the association (as it apparently is in masochism) or to the dissociation of the life and death drives? My personal answer is that, as with ambivalence, there are two ways of associating the life and death drives.

There is a primitive association in which the life and death drives are confused to the point of being indistinguishable, the one being sometimes mistaken for the other. That is the case with the drug addict and the masochist who confuse the life and death drives, sexual drives and self-destruction. They do not associate them because they do not distinguish them, they confuse them. I repeat what I have said in connection with the two forms of ambivalence: one cannot link what one has not previously distinguished. Whether it be under the aegis of the life drive or of the death drive or of the two mixed up together does not much matter; the result is the same: the drug addict destroys himself. This effect resembles one that may result from pre-genital oral ambivalence: it matters little to the subject whether it be through love or through hate that he is being devoured; all that counts as far as he is concerned is the result, namely that he is being eaten up.

By contrast, there is a more highly developed form of association in which the death and life drives are clearly distinguished, which makes it possible to link them together even while continuing to tell them apart. In that case, we do not confuse them but link up two distinct drives, which makes it possible to effect a life-enhancing synthesis between them. That is why I believe that this developed form of linking up the life and death drives underpins vital processes.

When patients fail to link the life and death drives, and in particular when they isolate or deny their death drive, then the vital processes are endangered. If the death drive is isolated instead of being combined with the life drive it can lead to destruction, and this the more so as, according to Freud, the death drives 'work essentially in silence' (Freud 1923a [1922]: 258) and are 'mute' (Freud 1923b: 59), which implies that the patient, unable to hear them, can neither curb them nor channel them to any good purpose. To illustrate the destructive effect of the separation of the drives I shall give an example taken from the analysis of Jack.

At the start of one session, Jack told me very proudly that to get to me in time he had driven through several red lights. When telling me that, he was focusing exclusively on his life drive, on his wish to be at the session, his affection for me. He did not see that such conduct was dangerous, that it expressed aggressive affects towards me and towards himself (aggressiveness turned back on himself through guilt) and a destructive force (auto- and hetero-destructiveness) as the psychic representative of the death drive. These psychic representatives of the death drive disturbed me all the more in that, no longer connected by Jack to his life drive, they escaped his vigilance: by disregarding the red lights, Jack was, in fact, all the more dangerous and vulnerable.

This blindness to danger illustrates the silent character of the work of the death drive: the patient does not hear or see that he has entered upon a destructive path. It may happen that as analysts we may feel tempted to behave as if we had not seen the destructive character of these activities, as if it were better not to draw the analysand's attention to this aspect in the hope that it would go away, but doing that would mean ignoring the strength of the drive. The analyst does far better to break the silence so that the patient can see the destructive character of what he is doing. It was only when I enabled Jack to take cognizance of his destructiveness and his aggressive affects that he was able, not to abandon them, but to look at them, to take them seriously, and to try to link them to his constructive tendencies, to place them in the service of life.

Does the danger of playing with vertigo depend more on the dissociation of the drives than on the difficulty of the game?

When they read about the exploits of Sylvain Saudan skiing down frozen couloirs, of Reinhold Messner climbing 8,000-metre peaks without oxygen, or of Philippe Petit walking a tightrope from the Chaillot Palace to the Eiffel Tower, many people think that the main pleasure these men take in playing with vertigo lies in the thrill of flirting with death. I believe that it is an infinitely more complex process, even if in isolated cases playing these vertiginous games hides a barely disguised suicidal tendency, akin to playing Russian roulette.

It must be borne in mind that those who take great risks while being fully aware of what they are doing play a far less dangerous game than those who take minimal risks without being aware of their own auto-destructive and hetero-destructive tendencies. Thus Jack would have been in a particularly dangerous situation had I not drawn his attention to his destructiveness. A man like Reinhold Messner, by contrast, is perfectly aware of the risks he runs and tries to face up to them; he portrays himself as a 'timid' mountaineer: 'If I were to overreach myself at 8,000 metres, I wouldn't survive!' (1980: 46). In his *Solo Nanga Parbat* he explains that he tries to anticipate all contingencies, to 'calculate down to the crevasses', to profit from the tiniest details of the experiences of those who have been there before him, to plan the best possible uphill routes and also to anticipate such inner dangers as the fits of panic liable to be evoked by solitude; finally he even foresees *that he cannot foresee everything*: 'I have mulled everything over, prepared everything, I am ready . . . I am determined to survive . . . I know that this climb is very dangerous and will push me to the limit of my capabilities. And there are many unavoidable dangers. And yet I leave nothing to chance' (*ibid.*: 141–3).

For the rest, all of us are surprised to discover that people who have survived the greatest dangers without ill effects may have a serious accident when the danger seems to be as good as gone. We often realize that when the accident happened the danger was not particularly great, but the person concerned was in a psychic state (guilt, sadness, grief, etc.) that favoured a disassociation of drives: he did not guard against the silent work of the destructive drive; he deliberately ignored the importance of his own self-destructive tendencies, which were then left uncurbed.

Messner is perfectly aware of the deadly risks he runs. Moreover, when he declared that he had lived through his own death several times and that he was thus able to discover that the fear of death disappears as it approaches, he recalled certain great thinkers, including Montaigne who, referring to the enemy that death seems to be, wrote in his *Essais*: 'Let us strip it of its strangeness, practise it, become used to it, let us bear nothing so much in mind as death' (1580, Book I, Chap. XX: 87). Messner also recalled what Montaigne wrote at the end of his life, when he saw death as the '*bout*' (end) and not the '*but*' (aim) of life: 'If we have not known how to live it is unjust to teach us how to die, and to wrench the end from the whole' (1580, Book III, Chap. XII). For all that, Messner, like those analysands who love to play dangerous games with vertigo, differ from such thinkers as Montaigne because they do not content themselves with reflections on death, but seem to seek the proximity of death in practice. In fact, Messner did not leave it at ideas and symbols; his knowledge also involved the body and the senses. 'The idea, the creation of an idea, is important to me. But without action, the idea is only half an idea. Every adventure in my life starts in my head, with a vision. But then I have to live it . . . I need the other half of the dream – action' (1989: 35).

The reason why I have quoted Messner at such length is that he clearly brings out the ambiguity of the questions raised by those patients who play dangerous games, games he manages to verbalize, while the patients – and it is perhaps for that very reason that they seek analysis – can only do so with great difficulty. Messner does not want to die, the proof being that he has come out alive from numerous situations that could have ended in his death; he wants to get as close to death as possible, but for all that he clings to life; I have the impression that he wants to come to know death while he is still alive. Now, during life it is impossible to come to know death personally, one can try to dream of it, to think of it, but not to experience it. Freud has said so, and many writers such as Thomas Mann have stressed it in their novels: 'So long as we are, death is not, and when death is present we are not. In other words, between death and us there is no rapport' (Mann 1928: 532).

Playing dangerous games with vertigo is not necessarily dicing with death

I think we must distinguish between analysands who dice with death and those who play dangerous games with vertigo. Now it is not death that the latter brave. The appearances may sometimes belie this fact and we may gain the impression that in both cases we are dealing with patients who take pleasure in facing death. In fact, the two cases are quite distinct.

The first, those who actually play with death, do not maintain a delicate balance between the life and death drives, and can be fitted into two groups. Either they confuse life drives with death drives and experience an eroticization of the death drive in the way drug addicts do. They do not constitute a separate group of analysands, but are 'vertigo junkies' much as some people are heroin junkies; it is quite possible that, like perverse patients, they are defending themselves against psychotic troubles in that way. Or else they dissociate the life and death drives and allow their destructive impulses to work in silence, unattached to Eros. These analysands do not constitute a separate group either. They are a part of that large group of analysands who, at one time or another, are unconscious of their destructive impulses. Like that large group, they are in great danger of being drawn to death unwittingly by their dissociated destructive impulses. And then there are the patients who play dangerous games with vertigo without there being any dissociation or confusion of drives; theirs is no longer a challenge to death. I believe that Sylvain Saudan, Reinhold Messner and Philippe Petit are men cast in the same mould; what they have to tell us can undoubtedly help us to understand what sometimes goes on in our analysands.

Why run such risks?

Defying death or defying one's limits?

Players of possible games rather than players of impossible games

Reinhold Messner gives me the impression of wishing to know death while he is still alive, and I think that this paradox accounts for something very important. Messner has no wish to die, but he does love to get as close as possible to the limit beyond which no more can be staked. One of his books, *Grenzbereich Todeszone* (1978), is aptly called *The Limit of Life* in translation. I think it is not death itself that interests those who play dangerous games with vertigo, but anything that tries to set them a *limit*, and moreover in all fields, even when that limit is of the most spectacular kind. The 'I shall go to the point where one can no longer live without oxygen' recalls the croupier's *rien ne va plus*, a call that can turn riches into poverty and vice versa in a moment.

This taste for testing one's limits is such that the limits must always be pushed further back as soon as they have been reached. No matter what the social level of those who play with vertigo, or the field in which they do so, it is obvious that the pleasure ceases once the limit has been reached; the continued attraction of the game then lies in the attempt to reach a new limit, beyond the one that has just been crossed. We see this quite clearly in the case of analysands who take more and more risky chances in their commercial or financial affairs, while calculating the financial risks just as meticulously as Messner prepares his Himalayan expeditions. Quite obviously it is not because they are pressed for money that they take these risks, since their personal fortune is often much greater than their lifestyle demands: their pleasure lies in constantly raising the vertiginous stakes.

Finally, what interests these *players with vertigo* is not the impossible but the possible, the 'How far can I go?' Messner put it as follows: 'I am seeking my "limits". I need to exceed my limits much as someone else needs drugs. Constantly. What I have reached so far interests me less. What I might (perhaps) reach now satisfies me, keeps me on my toes' (1989: 97). Sylvain Saudan has been called the skier of the impossible; I rather think that all these players should be called players of the possible. Their hankering after the limit seems to me a hankering after the fictitious zone in which the analysand experiences the two extremes that are combined in him and that he wants to keep together, such as strength and weakness, large and small, always and never, the knowable and the unknowable. Messner has tried to express how the fascination with the preparation of an expedition corresponds to his liking for the integration of extremes: 'To reduce the unforeseeable to the maximum and to live with the mystery despite everything. I know what awaits me but everything remains possible' (1980: 111).

Time as limit

Infinity is not eternity

Time is certainly a difficult limit to attain and also a source of vertigo. Hans Castrop, the hero of Thomas Mann's *The Magic Mountain*, succumbs to vertigo when he discovers a new flow of time that goes with life in the sanatorium:

> he would suddenly be overpowered by a mixture of terror and eager joy that made him fairly giddy. And this giddiness was in both senses of the word: rendering our hero not only dazed and dizzy, but flighty and light-headed, incapable of distinguishing between 'now' and 'then', and prone to mingle these together in a timeless eternity.
>
> (1928: 545)

This quotation underlines the problems of our patients torn between the repetition of the déjà vu (constancy of the object and of the ego) and of change, which brings us awareness of the passing of time.

But Thomas Mann opens up a frightful perspective: the magic of that sanatorium in the mountains saddles the hero with a monotonous idea of

161

time, in which nothing remarkable ever happens to give him what he calls an idea of being 'outside time' ('timeless eternity' in the English translation cited above). In fact, it gives him above all the illusion of infinite, that is endless, time, which must be distinguished from 'being outside time' (*hors du temps*), that is, from eternity. Time on the 'magic mountain' does indeed flow 'inside' time, it has a beginning and an end, namely death; but it seems to be endless because of its monotony, its repetitiveness and the passivity it arouses. It cannot, in my opinion, provide a positive perspective for the patient who constructs his own history during analysis, because it seems to be based on a confusion.

I believe that there is another view of eternity, one that is more fruitful in psychoanalysis. It involves the phantasy of a state of 'being outside time': beyond chronology, escaping from the notion of time flowing uniquely along a past–present–future track, a chronological vision evoking the illusion that the future can be pushed so far ahead that it borders on infinity. In this phantasy, we place ourselves 'outside time', that is leap into a different dimension, whence we can look down, at a single glance, on the whole of time, simultaneously taking in past, present and future without confusing them. This decentring effort may seem highly unusual but it is nevertheless an experience we have during intense moments, when we feel that we are being swept 'outside' the course of time and touch a new time dimension: the shock of beauty, of insight, of love are so many experiences allowing us to live, not in a time that never ends, but in what feels as if it were 'beyond' time. It is then that we come to know the meaning of eternity (being outside time) rather than of infinity (endless time). The poets may not be able to prove that it exists, but they give us an inkling of it:

> *Des milliers et des milliers d'années*
> *Ne sauraient suffir*
> *Pour dire*
> *La petite seconde d'éternité*
> *Où tu m'as embrassé*
> *Où je t'ai embrassée*
> *Un matin dans la lumière de l'hiver*
> *Au parc Monsouris à Paris*
> *À Paris sur la terre*
> *La terre qui est un astre.*
>
> (Jacques Prévert 1947–1949: 128)[1]

This view of eternity defies logic; yet some images or experiences can provide the elements for phantasies about it. Since the main subject of this book is vertigo, I should like to mention an image that has enabled one analysand to pass on from a spatial to a temporal idea, something moreover that helped him to gain a glimpse of eternity, as distinct from infinity.

This patient told me that he had reached a certain village on foot, that he had entered it, walked through it and then left it again. He had discovered this village chronologically, had seen successively and separately, first the way in, then the centre, and finally the way out. He could not envisage all three experiences simultaneously; all he could do was to linger in the centre of the village, believing that he would never be able to leave, that he would have to stay there for an infinity. Then he climbed up a hill overlooking the village, and at a single glance took in the way in, the centre and the way out. The three were distinct, spread out over a flat space, but visible all at once. He thought that eternity must be like that: without denying duration, he thought it possible to take in at a single glimpse of eternity all that happens in time.

In this phantasy of eternity, time – far from being denied – is acknowledged: an event has a beginning, runs its course, and comes to an end, but all three can be taken in at a glance because they are viewed from a different perspective; with the phantasies of infinity, by contrast, there is a denial of duration, as if there might be no end of time. Luc on top of the girder, in the grip of vertigo, had a phantasy of infinity, not of eternity.

Infinity causes vertigo

We are beginning to see how important the ideas of infinity and eternity may become in the course of an analysis. Many patients are gripped by vertigo when they think of the end of their analysis, because they are faced with two contradictory impulses hard to integrate. On the one hand, they would love the analysis to go on for ever, to be infinite; moreover unconsciously they often skip the last session before the vacation (they do not turn up, remain silent, or engage in idle chatter), behaving as if there were no last session and thus living out the illusion of infinity. But on the other hand, the idea of an endless analysis seems insupportable to them, negating as it does any idea of progress; nothing would matter any longer: why say something that you have 'all your life' to say? These patients find that infinity fills them with anxiety, while the zest for life is bound up with the appreciation of life's ephemeral nature. The patient who supplied the image of the village seen from the top of a hill concluded: 'An analysis that would never end would be sheer paradise . . .'. Then, suddenly: ' . . . but a paradise without an end, what horror!' He might equally well have said: 'A life without end, what horror!'

When a patient discovers the phantasy of eternity he takes a quite different view of the end of his analysis. He may consider maintaining within him a living analysis with a beginning, a development and an end, embedded in time but preserved in an eternal dimension. For the analysand we have just mentioned the phantasy of an infinite life was frightening because it involved the denial of a human dimension, namely time, which lends shape to life; but the phantasy of eternity is something quite different because, far

163

from denying a human dimension, it adds a new one, one we can imagine even it is not naturally given to us – much as men could imagine, without being birds, what it is like to negotiate three-dimensional space and invent aeroplanes and similar flying machines.

I believe some patients try to have experiences leading them to ideas that help them to get close to this view of eternity. What my patient was able to make explicit in his view from the hill, other patients seek unconsciously in different situations, for instance by climbing mountain peaks to 'see things from above', or by listening to music that makes them feel the beauty of a great work behind the succession of notes but without forgetting about them, or again by looking at nature.

An analysand told me at the end of her analysis, when she found herself in a very sad situation and was being torn apart by the conflicting decisions she had to make: 'I shall try to reach for the stars'. What she meant was that she would try to 'get off' the chronological plane, off the ground, to rise up and look down on things as she might in the light of eternity. This was not a piece of madness, but a creative act, one that enabled her, even while the road seemed blocked, to try to invent a way out by daring to create a new dimension in phantasy.

Analysands try to reach an internal object by playing these dangerous games

Some characteristics of this internal object

All analysands who play these dangerous games with vertigo in some specific way have always struck me as being engaged in a quest apparently shared by all of them: they brave danger not for its own sake but because it characterizes the problem involved in meeting the object they wish to know. The downhill slope, the snow, the mountain and the air may be treated by these analysands, lovers of dangerous games, like living persons, dangerous and fascinating, whom they desperately need to know. It often seems obvious to me that through these games they are, in fact, trying to reach quite another object, namely an internal one that may be their mother, or any other person important to them, one whom they are trying to define. With the help of these natural obstacles they thus hope to gain a more precise and tangible idea of this elusive internal object.

This object causes anxiety because it is fuzzy and elusive

Danger brings out the anxiety this object gives rise to. The analysand does not fear the void, in which he might break his neck, but the object which

164

he has a vital need to know. That object can be frightening because it eludes him and is therefore undefinable. Hence it is the more frightening the more difficult it is to plumb. I even believe that the reason why death sometimes seems to be the object the analysand wants to know, is not that he wants to know death itself, but above all because it is the classic example of an object impossible to know, since no human being has ever been able to experience it personally. As Freud put it, the unconscious lacks any representation of death because we have no memory traces of what we have not experienced.

Does this object seem frightening at times because it is forbidden?

For a very long time, Philippe Petit, the tightrope walker, had dreamed of walking between the towers of Notre-Dame in Paris on a tightrope, and knowing that the police had set their face against it, he went ahead with it all the same knowing perfectly well that he would be arrested. As he put it, he would thus get the 'state of weightlessness' to rub shoulders with the 'state of arrest' (1991: 182). I believe that I would be inhaling incestuous perfume and defying any who dared to forbid it, were I to treat myself to a symbolic reading of Petit's text, a text so rich in sensory discoveries, especially so in the following passage: 'Equilibrium is voluptuous. Notre-Dame belongs to me, Paris belongs to me, the vast sky belongs to me, it makes me forget to breathe' (*ibid.*: 183).

A fascinating object

The gravity of the danger incurred also brings out the immensity of the analysand's need to get to know this object. One of its characteristics is precisely that it is perilous to know, but also fascinating and magnificent. Perhaps once known it may turn out to be less frightening and less fascinating?

An object that must be grasped with the help of the senses

To get to know this object, those analysands who play dangerous games with vertigo need to sense it: they need to feel it, not merely to know it through their thoughts or phantasies; thoughts and phantasies are indeed involved but must ceaselessly be checked against corporeal knowledge. Philippe Petit speaks with great emotion of the vivid and sensual way in which he discovers the air when he advances high up on his rope, lost in space: 'No one must hear, no one must know that my heart is beating, that it is beating so slowly, that it has stopped beating, that my senses have multiplied tenfold, that my nose gathers in the scattered molecules of the air, that I become intoxicated with perfumes, that I invent colours . . . No one must suspect that as I advance along the rope, my lips taste the sugary breeze, that I progress through sweetmeats' (1991: 96–7). And further on he adds: 'I inhale the heights, I taste the depths, I breathe in the wind and the air' (*ibid*.: 164).

Can we say that the mountains, the snow, the air, the sea, the vastness, and so on, *are* the frightening and fascinating unknown object these analysands wish to reach? Or should we rather say that they *replace* it? That they *represent* it? Even *symbolize* it? I cannot give a general answer; there are only personal ones. Let me simply say that the more I tend to use the verb *to be* in my answer, the more I voice the fear that the game is dangerous; and the more willing I am to use the verb *to symbolize* the less I fear the game.

What object has to be found? A mother capable of reverie

Here we are back with the *nameless dread* first mentioned in Chapter 2 because, even if it is impossible to make generalizations about all the players of impossible games, I have found a common link in all those I have had in analysis: in the course of their analysis they have all expressed the need to repeat the experience of a nameless dread they experienced at an early age. That age, before the emergence of speech, explains moreover why they should have felt the need for such repetition and why my interpretations involve the understanding and recall of a sensory and corporeal experience, that is, involve infraverbal communication leading to verbalization.

These analysands discovered, in the course of their analysis, that they had experienced, during the first few months of their lives, a sensation of dying that they could not work over at the time with the help of the mother's capacity for reverie. The reconstruction, during analysis, of the history of every one of these analysands made it clear that their mother herself had such great fears that her beloved child might die that she was unable to contain the child's anxiety, or even to realize that the child was anxious. The child was thus left with a meaningless and hence unassimilable dread. In some cases, however, it seems that the mother would have been able to accept her child's anxiety had not the child, because of his envy, disabled her capacity for reverie.

In analysis, these patients repeat in various ways the occasions giving rise to nameless dread: they continue to do so until the analyst takes cognizance of the fact that they look upon him in the transference as a mother robbed of her capacity for reverie. Before these patients can find their own way of assigning a meaning to their anxiety, they must first be enabled to express their aggressiveness towards their beloved mother-analyst whom, in the transference, they hold very dear, but also consider to be lacking in the capacity for reverie, and, moreover, be helped to realize that the reason why they keep repeating their nameless dread in the analysis is to discover its meaning in it with the analyst's help. They have a need to construct an internal object capable of understanding them, the better to discover their own capacity for understanding. To do that, these patients must, I believe, be able to combine their feeling that their mother had failed them at a very anxious moment in their life, with trust that she will nevertheless take good care of them and that, in contact with her, they may discover their own ability to take care of themselves.

A 'white-ceiling mother'

To illustrate the various ways in which an analysand can unconsciously communicate his nameless dread to the analyst, I shall now say a few words about Jane. During the preliminary interviews, Jane told me at length about her anxiety and anger at the dangerous games of others: a child who kept balancing on a window ledge in order to taunt her, or an adult who black-mailed her with the threat of suicide. At the time she thus presented herself as a person preoccupied with her own anxiety triggered off by the danger-ous actions of others. Once the analysis had started, the roles were reversed. It was Jane who now played dangerous games with vertigo, taking enormous risks or threatening to take them in such a way that I felt deeply anxious about her. Moreover, on the couch, she had fits of vertigo of various types: fusion-related vertigo with a fear of self-destruction; suction-related vertigo during which she struggled to tear apart the phantasy chains that kept her prisoner on the couch, and imprisonment/escape-related vertigo coupled to an urge to walk out of the consulting room despite the wish that I hold her back. In my counter-transference I had the continuous impression that I was close to the void, because it looked as if Jane might break off the analysis at any moment and that we were teetering on the brink of an abyss.

Then came a session when I fully took stock of the feelings associated with my counter-transference, and this marked a turning point in the analy-sis. I realized that Jane had to make me feel the pull of the abyss lest I abandon her in her effort not to fall into it. That session started with a long silence filled with anxiety which I finally broke with a throaty growl meant simply to let her know that I was there, present. Jane then said to me, 'How can you expect me to talk with that white ceiling on top of me!' I was completely taken aback: the ceiling of my consulting room is not white. In effect, Jane was talking about the ceiling of her inner world: about the projection of the frightening internal object she wanted to get to know and which had always eluded her.

I was aware of the polysemy of 'white', and did not wish to break the thread of Jane's associations let alone insinuate my own. And so I simply asked 'What's a white ceiling feel like to you?' I did not ask 'What is that?', because I did not want to press her for a ready-made or reifying answer. By asking 'What's it *like*?', I thought I was addressing Jane's emotions, bringing home to her the originality of anyone looking at the qualities of the object in the light of the significance he attributes to it and the context in which he places it. Her answer came at once, 'All hospital ceilings are white, I feel here as if I were in the hospital bed . . . Oh! But your ceiling isn't white! This is the first time I noticed that!' Later, I said to her, 'You said, the hospital bed, as if you were thinking of a particular hospital'. Once again the reply came straightaway, 'It can only be the hospital where I was taken some weeks after my birth.'

Jane thus tried, by linking her current feelings to the stories told her by her family, to reconstruct a dramatic hospitalization experience she had had as a baby: her feeling that she was being kept on the couch as she had been in the hospital bed where she had been given blood transfusions, the isolation, her mother's anxiety, the impression that everything was out to hurt her, but above all her sense of being completely incapable of understanding what was happening to her and what she was experiencing. It was not so much her history as such that was important for her to rediscover as the links between it and her present life, the persistence of her undefined anxiety in the present, and the need to repeat it by playing dangerous games, in analysis and outside, until her anxiety began to make sense. The white ceiling thus became the representation of a mother incapable of making sense of what Jane was experiencing.

This was a crucial turning point in the analysis, because Jane had been able to make me feel that I was, in the transference, that white-ceiling mother who had proved incapable of helping her to think straight: while I remained that mother unaware of my incapacity for reverie, Jane could not, in fact, tell me anything, because she did not understand anything. The paradox involved in the counter-transference was obvious: I had to feel my incapacity to understand Jane's anxiety in the counter-transference, and to agree to take it into account, so as to give proof of my capacity for reverie. I thus discovered what my feeling that I had an incapacity for reverie meant in the counter-transference. It was essential that my capacity for reverie allow me to interpret myself in the transference as a mother devoid of a capacity for reverie, before Jane could supply me with the means of grasping the image of the white-ceiling mother she carried within her as an internal object beyond her comprehension. And it was only when she herself was able to envisage her internal object, the white-ceiling mother, that she could appreciate that I was different: 'Oh! Your ceiling isn't white!', thus creating the indispensable differentiation in space needed for the emergence of symbolism.

We then began to realize that Jane was trying, in her games with vertigo, to achieve more than the repetition of a frightening situation she was trying to understand; she was also trying to find a mother who would not leave her with that nameless anxiety. That very primitive mother was difficult to define; she was naturally confused with the frightening situation as such as well as with Jane. That is why Jane, by resorting to vertigo in an attempt to escape from it, was somehow behaving as if she were trying to discover her own capacity for understanding the anxiety even while attempting to extricate herself from it; and also to discover her mother's capacity for understanding Jane's anxiety and to help her get rid of it. In such cases, the material triggering the anxiety (the white ceiling) may itself be a mental image of the mother to be rediscovered (a white-ceiling mother). This seems to be the case especially when analysands presenting vertigo give one the impression that they are treating the sea, the earth, the mountains or the air as so many persons.

In other fields, too, for instance political, financial, scientific, artistic and commercial affairs, every experience of vertigo can fill these patients with the hope of coming up with a slightly better definition of that fascinating and intangible internal object: their mother unable to exercise her capacity for reverie.

Defying the limit: vertigo or equilibrium?

When a player of impossible games meets an impassable threshold, for instance a physiological threshold that is objectively insuperable, he often seeks another field in which he can try to challenge fresh limits, and so avoid running the graver risks. This, I believe, is one of the major themes of Luc Besson's film *The Big Blue* in which the hero, having dived as far down as he can without strapping on an aqualung prefers to die rather than stop at that limit. In effect, the player of impossible games has a vital need to push the limits further out and to continue to get ever closer to the unknowable; hence, when he comes up against an impassable limit it becomes vitally important for him to have the unknowable assume a different face, so that he may continue his attempts to get closer to it.

With these particular problems posed by the players of impossible games we are back with what has been at the back of our remarks about the search for equilibrium associated with the various forms of vertigo. Those who challenge their limits without running too many risks have de-idealized these limits as well as the challenge they issue to them. They can accordingly grant themselves the pleasure of taking measured 'doses' of the challenge. This de-idealization often occurs when, in analysis, the patient realizes how important it is for him to hanker after what he does not possess or cannot do, even while realizing how essential it is to have limits, to go short of things and to have wishes. The de-idealization of limits enables the analysand to find some meaning in the challenge he issues to them. It is then that he tastes the pleasure of brushing up against the limit, and is no longer afraid of doing so.

One of the most fascinating limits for players of impossible games is often the imaginary limit between life and death. It may happen that in the course of their analysis patients begin to conceive of death as a limit inherent in life, as an intrinsic part of it, and as something that lends meaning to life: 'Death is a decisive moment in this life. It is not something that happens at the end of our life like a scream; it is like a pole that confers tension to our existence' (Messner 1989: 212). Like Messner, the analysand who thought 'a life without end, what horror!' was making a comment on the importance of the ephemeral aspect of human existences: 'Death gives my life a clearly-defined direction. My life is limited. I know that I shall die. And because I know it, I live intensely' (*ibid.*: 191). And so the analysand can go in search of equilibrium, daring to taste the pleasure of having life-enriching experiences, even if they entail a risk. He is again in the grip of two conflicting tendencies: living without any risks and hence constricting his existence, and taking ill-considered risks which means despising life. As always, the equilibrium towards which he tends, and which can be a source of pleasure, is not the precise middle between the total absence and a surfeit of risks: this equilibrium involves the original creation of a way that allows for both personal growth and the running of risks. This creation integrates two conflicting tendencies and is accompanied by a sense of pleasure.

The quest for a creation that integrates conflicting aspirations goes hand in hand with the search for an object endowed with a capacity for reverie; it is a quest filled with hate and love at one and the same time. In fact, for an analysand to embark on a creative but dangerous exploit can be an aggressive reproduction of the danger he felt his mother had left him to face all by himself once upon a time; it is therefore an auto-aggressive and hetero-aggressive attack. But at the same time it can also be a way of checking whether he can extricate himself from frightening situations, and hence of proving to himself that he has internalized a mother capable of lending a meaning and finding an answer to frightening situations. In demonstrating his own capacity to solve what lies at the limit of the possible, he tells himself again that the frightening situation he is repeating, and in which his beloved mother's capacity for reverie was wanting, was a violent and difficult one, but at the same time he can prove to himself that, though his mother has cruelly failed him, he can by his own efforts render her present and restore her, because in proving his own capacities he can demonstrate that he has introjected her despite everything: both her and her capacity to take care of him.

The reason why I stress the specific nature of vertigo is that the dangerous game played with it by many analysands involves attempts to avoid it by trying to decrease the gap between their two internal voices, one in the register of omnipotence, and the other in the register of realistic power and hence critical of the first. However, the method the analysand uses to decrease the gap between his two internal voices is odd: he tries to demonstrate that his triumph which might appear to be of an omnipotent kind, is nothing of the kind, that it is not in the least magical, that, in his case, it is a feasible achievement, and hence one falling into the realm of realistic power. The game then consists in administering very fine doses of the difficult exploit, to place it precisely at the limit where what appeared to be impossible (only achievable by the magic of omnipotence) proves to be possible for the player all the same.

The meticulous way of determining that dose shows clearly that it is the result of an integrative force aimed at combining the infantile, omnipotent part with the evolved part of the self, thus demonstrating that what was taken for omnipotence was nothing of the kind. Philippe Petit, for instance, was able to prove that walking from the Trocadero to the Eiffel Tower on a tightrope was not a magical feat. However, in order to prove that, he had to determine his point of arrival very finely: he attached his rope just under the second storey of the Tower; had he attached it a few centimetres higher, the final slope would have been too steep and he would never have managed to get across. For these players of impossible games, the game with vertigo consists in not having vertigo. It seems plain, in fact, that if they do not have vertigo it is because they design their game very carefully instead of seeking illusory magical victories likely to let them down; they aim for triumphs that are both spectacular and attainable: that is, brilliant but in no way magical.

I would liken these exploits, performed with a cool head, to the feats of somnambulists. Claire Degoumois, who has made a study of somnambulism, stresses that sleep-walkers never fall, even when they engage in the most impossible acrobatic feats. This makes me think that they resemble our adventurers into the impossible inasmuch as their exploits, however spectacular, are feasible. In fact, sleep-walkers, like our adventurers, seem to keep their feet on the ground: they may walk across roofs but do not try to take off. Like those engaged on impossible adventures, they therefore know how to administer just the right doses of what is attainable in the realm of the grandiose; but the important difference is that their dosage, instead of being the result of a deliberate calculation, is administered without their conscious control, thus depriving them of the pleasure of realizing that the exploit is of their own making. For Claire Degoumois, the sleep-walker resembles someone who cannot carry off an exploit unless propped up by the power of his parents; she speaks of sleep-walkers as 'divested of their own will to control their mobility, filled only with the active power of their parents' (1992). By contrast, analysands who play dangerous games with vertigo have a keen perception of their personal capacities and limitations; they try to use them as best they can. While sleep-walkers perform their feats without fear but wake up feeling ashamed, the second group feel fear during their exploits as a counterpoint to their pleasure.

Note

1 Thousands and thousands of years / Would not suffice / To tell / The small second of eternity / When you kissed me / When I kissed you / One morning in the light of winter / In Monsouris Park in Paris / In Paris on the earth / On the earth which is a heavenly body.

Equilibrium: a continuous construction

The idea of vertigo involves that of equilibrium, but it should be remembered, as I have tried to explain in Chapter 10, that in moving on from the first idea to the second we are also changing our mode of discourse. Vertigo appears because of the conflict between two inner voices which the analysand cannot reconcile since they are in different keys. Equilibrium, on the other hand, corresponds to an integrating voice trying to combine contraries that are integrable because they are in the same key – the feeling of disequilibrium appears when the analysand prefers one of the contraries to the other. I believe that the search for equilibrium is inseparable from the study of vertigo, because it reflects an integrating tendency of the analysand to surmount his vertigo, and because it takes over from vertigo to the extent that the analysand manages to reduce the split between his omnipotent infantile attitude and his more highly developed attitude.

Equilibrium is not the happy medium between smallness and immensity

Is the search for equilibrium a sign of timidity?

What I have been saying about the renunciation of the omnipotence of the ego, of that of the object and of that of their relationship, and also what we have noted during the transition from the unlimited narcissistic world to a world with limits, might have given the reader the mistaken impression that vertigo is simply the result of too grandiose a view of the world or of oneself. As if, on reading 'The eternal silence of these infinite spaces frightens me' (*Pensées*, n.d.: No. 206), we concluded that Pascal, instead of trying to convey awe in the face of such immensity, were merely advising us not to look too far ahead and so to keep our balance. Actually, the problem of those trying to find their balance is to realize that, in one and the same register, namely that of potency, we are both very small and infinitely great – so many specks of dust reaching up to the stars thanks to their psychic faculties – instead of renouncing either dimension, allowing ourselves to be torn apart between the two, or falling into the void constituting the space between them.

Our infantile part hankers after magical omnipotence because the feeling that we are weak is so intense that it may become unbearable. Now, renouncing our infantile omnipotence does not mean renouncing the immense, genuinely powerful aspect of ourselves and being left with our smallness alone. On the contrary, it means holding on to both aspects – smallness and immensity – but stripped of their magical character; while the hankering after omnipotence implies that in order to retain the magical sense of our own or the object's immensity we must disregard their smallness.

Is equilibrium the happy medium?

The analysand finds it hard to see how he might arrive at balance while preserving the sense of smallness *and* of the immensity of the *I*, of the *object* and of their relationship: as soon as he leans towards either smallness or immensity, the feeling of disequilibrium suddenly appears, because favouring either tendency means forfeiting the other dimension of oneself.

It is clear that the solution based on the attempt to strike a balance halfway between the two – neither too great nor too small – would prove very disappointing, because it would mean settling for a happy medium that, while not causing vertigo, entails a form of immobility, whereas real balance is always shifting and in need of being restored. Some of my patients were loath to start analysis because they feared that it might lead them to enjoy a happy medium that would render them mediocre, rob them of their genius; one patient said that she did not wish to 'turn grey' even if that would make her happier. She came to realize gradually that, in analysis, it is never a question of mixing black and white to produce grey, but of keeping the two colours distinct by linking them; what is flat may be uniformly grey, but the moment there is volume the simultaneous presence of distinct dark and bright parts sets both of them off.

It is no more satisfying to imagine equilibrium based on hovering between the two dimensions. This seems to be reflected in some of Chagall's paintings where a man seems torn between his feet rooted in the earth while his arms are being drawn towards the sky by a woman or an angel.

Nor can greater balance be attained by attempts to close the gap between the two extremes until they touch and merge with each other. If man's immensity and smallness are treated as similar qualities, the result is disequilibrium once again. Milan Kundera makes this point in *The Unbearable Lightness of Being*; he relates that Stalin's son committed suicide when the British officers with whom he had been interned in Germany during the Second World War remonstrated with him for leaving the latrines in a filthy state and forced him to clean them out. He succumbed to vertigo because he, Stalin's son and hence the Son of God, had been judged, not for something sublime, but 'for shit':

> Were the very highest of drama and the very lowest so vertiginously close? Vertiginously close? Can proximity cause vertigo? It can. When the north pole comes so close as to touch the south pole, the earth disappears and man finds himself in a void that makes his head spin and beckons him to fall. If rejection and privilege are one and the same, if there is no difference between the sublime and the paltry, if the son of God can undergo judgment for shit, then human existence loses its dimensions and becomes unbearably light.
>
> (Kundera 1985: 244)

Equilibrium: an exit towards the top

Victor Hugo summed up the drama of *Ruy Blas* in a famous metaphor: 'An earthworm in love with a star' (1838: 1594). Ruy Blas was torn between his earthworm pole and his star pole; at given moments he tried to forget one or other, and in the end he died from attempting to combine the two by confusing them. This search for a possible way out between the two extremes is the main theme of Victor Hugo's book, every one of its tragic characters trying to find a way of combining within him extremes he believes to be irreconcilable; this search for equilibrium, and moreover the evocation of vertigo, touches each one of us and remains so topical that Victor Hugo's tragedy is as relevant today as ever it was in the past. But Ruy Blas found no way out; he died, much as Stalin's son died in Kundera's book.

The analysand in search of equilibrium generally realizes during his analysis that there can be no possible confusion of an earthworm with a star, and that there can be no happy medium between the two, and that there is no call to renounce either of them. In fact, most often, patients discover through analysis that there is one way out, a way that emerges thanks to the opening up of a new dimension: the analysand can effect, within himself, a synthesis of these two dimensions – smallness and immensity – by integrating them in the unique person that happens to be himself. As long as he can only imagine a single line leading from smallness to immensity, he is bound to feel unbalanced, because he is either impoverished by the abandonment

175

of one of the extremes, torn between the two, or paralysed by their confusion. I believe that the search for equilibrium entails leaving the linear level for another dimension, namely that of creation or generation, the better to integrate the smallness and the immensity in the creation of the *I* and of the *object*. The patient then tries to create a path on which he can combine his feelings of being so small that he still has everything to learn, but so large that he transcends the limits of a quantifiable world: a drop of water thinking of the ocean.

Some people owe their fame to creations that bring out this synthesis in a spectacular way: Beethoven was at the mercy of his defective hearing, but he nevertheless wrote music that opened up a world of beauty, beyond anything quantifiable. Our patients sometimes confront us with very simple creations that achieve this synthesis between smallness and immensity in the everyday world: one of my patients, a mother, was profoundly aware of the infinitely precious and unquantifiable affection she conveyed to her children in the slices of bread and butter with jam she prepared. She created equilibrium by linking, in a synthesis, the very simple act of feeding with an affective force that was not measurable but infinitely precious, the first needing the second to express itself while endowing it with meaning.

A progression imposed by solitude; the de-idealization of equilibrium

Believing that you are in balance is as good as having lost it

One of the paradoxes of the search for equilibrium lies in the fact that, to enjoy a degree of it, we have to accept that we can never fully attain it; in effect, since equilibrium has to be perpetually created, it is gone as soon as it has been attained. Equilibrium calls for constant readjustment because it is an incessant search for harmonious relations between a developing ego and a constantly changing environment, communicating through an external and an internal space which they help to create. The discovery of this interaction, combining space and time, goes hand in hand with the ability to keep oneself afloat, with buoyancy, which presupposes introjective identification with an object sufficiently reliable and itself endowed with an uplifting capacity, together with the experience of solitude.

No one can live my life for me

If he is to assuage his normal apprehension and to attain equilibrium, the analysand cannot dispense with personal experience, so much so that at the last moment, when all the conditions combine to allow him to surmount his vertigo, he must still clear the hurdle of such experience. It is rather like the courage the novice swimmer needs the first time he lets go of the edge of the pool: 'Everything tells me that I shall float on the surface but if I sink, it's me who will be sinking!' It is also like the courage needed by the mountaineer to let go of the rock face during his first abseiling attempt, or more simply of the small child who lets go of the adult's hand for the first time to take its first unaided steps. I was struck by the courage it took Luc to unclasp the hand clinging to analysis. He should have seen the end of that long analysis coming well before he actually did, but while he knew rationally that he could now develop further on his own, he had an almost physical resistance to abandoning immobility for the experience of moving in time and space, where equilibrium is gained by the concatenation of unstable positions. He found it hard to really believe that was possible before having taken the risk of trying it out in the solitude of personal experience.

Every one of us has taken this leap into the void of personal experience at some time in his life, because it goes with the discovery of solitude. Every one of us has had one of those moments that face us with the incontrovertible evidence that our life cannot be lived by anyone else, and that no one else can have this ineluctable experience in our place. 'Often these are moments when the corporeal aspect of the ego is highlighted, during physical illness for example, but also during pregnancy with certain women: "Now that this baby is in my womb it has of course to come out, I shall be forced to go through the experience of childbirth; and though I cannot tell in advance what that experience will be like, I shall be forced to experience it for myself." . . . but of course one of the most crucial moments for the patient, when he is most prone to this anxiety of being left alone, is when he is faced with the proximity of his own death' (D. Quinodoz 1991a: 31).

Much the same thing happens when someone dear to us goes through an unhappy time and is left to cope with it all on his own, when we would so like to change places with him and so spare him the pain; this is particularly true of parents whose children have a very painful experience; they then realize that their child will have to bear this suffering all by himself and that all their love for him cannot help him to avoid it. They have given him life and now that life is his own for better or for worse, and no one can live it on his behalf.

There are also moments when solitude involves a purely emotional experience, for instance when a patient has to make a crucial choice and realizes that he has just one life, that choosing one thing means renouncing the rest for ever, and that he alone can make the choice that will determine the only life he has to live.

This acceptance of solitude is also part of the pursuit of equilibrium, because it is linked to the de-idealization of one's own or of the object's omnipotence. Thus, at the start of his psychoanalysis, Luc refused to pay a hospital visit to a relative of whom he was very fond and who had just had a major operation: 'I can do nothing to relieve him, so what good would my going to see him do? What would I be doing there?' At the end of his analysis, Luc was amazed at his former attitude, because he had come to realize that, even if it was not effective, his presence might have been important - indeed, the very acceptance of his helplessness might have brought the patient some relief.

Inventing one's life as one goes along

The construction of equilibrium also involves the solitary process of inventing one's own life. This is what Nils discovered. Nils was an analysand very good at dressing in other people's clothes and at slipping into the thoughts of others, which he was able to express very well; moreover he loved to be on the stage. However, he suffered a great deal from not feeling that he was himself; he had the impression that he was going through life playing a part that was not his; he no longer knew which were his own feelings or his own thoughts. In the course of his analysis, Nils had begun to have dizzy spells, to feel unsteady on his feet. This happened at a time when he became aware of the loneliness inherent in the feeling of being oneself: he could no longer think what he ought to be thinking; he had to decide that for himself. The fear of loneliness went hand in hand with the fear of daring to think thoughts that might well be greeted with derision. However, not feeling himself thinking his own thoughts was even worse.

It was then that Nils told me a dream, the material of which served as a representation and symbol for understanding his fear of loneliness, helping us to get rid of his symptoms of vertigo. In that dream, Nils was acting in a play and discovered to his dismay that he had not learned his lines; the other actors were playing their parts, the audience was listening, but he did not know what he was expected to say. It was appalling – he had not even read the play. Moreover, he was furious with the prompter who failed to come to his aid. Nils started by telling me that the whole thing was like his analysis, thus giving voice to his anger at my failure to prompt him how to live; he had thought that an analyst would show him how to conduct his life, but I did not invariably tell him how to play his role. I then drew his attention to the fact that it was he himself who had produced the dream in which he did not know his lines and in which no one had prompted him. Might he perhaps be satisfying an unconscious wish in that way? Since Nils failed to understand what I was getting at, I tried to be more specific. 'Perhaps you used to think until now', I said, 'that your life was a part written out in advance and that I, the prompter, must have read it, and hence would know all the answers in advance as well. In your dream, you may well be granting a wish, of which you have not been aware until now, namely the wish to invent your own role in life as you go along.' My suggestion had an astonishing effect, because Nils had been sure that I would blame him for being a bad pupil who held everyone else back because he had not learned his lines; he said that he had even deflected his guilt about being a bad pupil on to the prompter who did not tell him his part.

Nils was staggered when he suddenly remembered the sequel to this dream: after his first panic, he had gone on to dream that he managed perfectly well on the stage and was astonished at his ability to invent his lines as he went along. The audience and his fellow actors looked as if they found the whole thing perfectly normal. All I myself had to add therefore was, 'Deep down, you are utterly surprised to realize that your role in life has not been written out in advance and that you alone can invent it as you go along.'

The symptom of vertigo disappeared. The ideas suggested by the dream, such as improvising his role, producing his own lines instead of waiting for someone else to prompt him as to what to say, were able from then on to serve Nils as so many landmarks; he appreciated the symbolic bearing these ideas might have on his own creativity: the solitude he was forced to endure to think his own thoughts was offset by the positive feeling that he himself was alive. The part he played in his dream now symbolized his life, which he invented without the need for a dress rehearsal, and whose meaning he would not be able to fathom until he had spoken his last lines. As a result of his newly won creativity, Nils had come to realize that the sense of inner stability and equilibrium was linked to the flow of his life: taking the leap of improvising his own life, his very own life, rather than believing that he must rattle off the lines of a sublime life, also meant being content not to know, here and now, what lines he would be speaking tomorrow.

Here we have an example of the idea of change in continuity being applied by the analysand to himself and no longer to his objects: he knows that he will remain *himself*, even though he cannot tell at any one moment how he will act in the next scene. His reaction may well take him by surprise. The willingness to be surprised by himself depends on the analysand's certainty of remaining himself; this willingness is complementary to the capacity to remain surprised by the object despite its constancy. Such surprise at a perpetual development is a guarantee against boredom despite one's own and the object's constancy; this constancy, in its turn, being the guarantee against anxiety despite the surprises that the constant development of oneself and of the object holds in store for us all.

The personal experience of equilibrium: a leap into the void

Even when the internal and external conditions seem joined to banish the feeling of vertigo, the symptom may persist. This is because the road to the personal experience of leaping into the void of solitude is still blocked. Some people have no difficulty in clearing it, and their vertigo disappears by itself during analysis: as the psychoanalytic process keeps unfolding by way of the analysand's associations, the analysand comes to realize one fine day that he no longer has vertigo. For others, such as Luc, the analysis must be continued until the removal of the obstacle to that difficult personal experience; this may involve the realization that the apparent danger underlying vertigo must not be mistaken for a real threat. The patient may retain an intense reflex anxiety about internal and external dangers, even though he no longer relates these to terrifying phantasies. He must have the courage to believe that a difference is possible not only between his impression and external reality, but also between that impression and his inner reality. What matters is to know the difference between the impression of danger, which is a real enough impression, and the actual internal and external threat. Now, being able to tell that difference calls for personal experience, which comes back to realizing that 'it is I myself who am going through all this, and no one else in my stead'.

Waiting for the right moment

In an earlier chapter we saw that Luc had this kind of personal experience when he climbed up a ladder to show the way to a colleague. He knew that the ladder was solid, he had moreover analysed his phantasies linked to competition-related vertigo, and he no longer had an internal reason for having vertigo on that ladder. Furthermore, he had been able to discover in his analysis that there can be a difference between the intensity of a sensation or a feeling and the gravity of what it relates to: someone might, for instance, complain of a very bad pain even if it is caused by a minor complaint. Luc still needed the personal experience of braving a situation likely to give him vertigo before he could be sure that he no longer suffered from it. That occasion was provided by a colleague who asked Luc for direction.

Admittedly, when the external and internal conditions do not combine to prevent the emergence of vertiginous anxiety, the personal experience of a 'leap into the void' may strengthen the patient's defences; if someone does not make the right swimming strokes or clings to the phantasy of being absorbed by an internal object symbolized for him by the bottom of the pool, he would do well not to torture himself with the wish to let go at the deep end of the pool; were he to do so suddenly in these circumstances, he would sink. On the other hand, when the conditions are such that the feeling of vertigo does not appear, or that the danger heralded by the feeling of vertigo does not materialize, it is still essential that the analysand discover by personal experience that, notwithstanding his apprehensions, there is no real danger or that the threat is negligible.

The deconditioning of vertigo

The reason why I dwell on the personal experience of leaping into the void is that some people have been able to rid themselves of vertigo, especially of vertigo associated with climbing mountains or with air travel, by special training or deconditioning. Like Skopek and Carreras (1988), I have been able to observe that for some people this meant making quite certain that the real danger is negligible, being well informed about all the contingencies that might arise, and also about the best way of dealing with them; and thus de-dramatizing the situation. After that, they still had to take a leap into the void, for which an emotionally propitious context – say the company of like-minded people – is essential.

We see that in this form of deconditioning none of the unconscious reasons that might have elicited the vertigo is taken into consideration and that this is therefore no kind of psychoanalysis. These techniques can be applied, above all in cases of mountain vertigo, or in those cases of vertigo of somatic, non-pathological, origin, which I mentioned in Chapter 1; those affected can be taught to correct the data supplied by their sensory system or at least take them into consideration. As for patients suffering from vertigo of psychic origin, such deconditioning methods may simply displace their symptom for another, less unpleasant, one. In my view, these methods are useful mainly for persons who have remained stuck with a symptom that appeared at a given moment of their life as the expression of a temporary inner conflict. Once the conflict had passed, the alarm system kept ringing, the condition for turning it off being that the person concerned have the personal experience I have called leaping into the void.

Between vertigo and equilibrium: playing with space and time, the changeable and the immutable, instantaneity and duration

Moving equilibrium vs. vertigo due to immobility

Patients suffering from vertigo often liken equilibrium to immobility, and vertigo to movement. They feel rather as if, thanks to their analysis, they can 'discover' equilibrium, and can then go on to 'maintain' it statically, behaving as if 'at last they can sit in an armchair without budging, just like the analyst'. At that point they have not the least suspicion that the analyst feels far from immobile in his armchair, but is constantly busy readjusting his balance. Later, they discover the paradox, that equilibrium goes hand in hand with the deployment of movements in space and time, while vertigo goes hand in hand with frozen immobility. I come back to the image that helped to enlighten Luc at the end of his analysis: 'When I balance on a swing, I can go as high as the swing will go without danger, but if I stop the swing at the top, I shall fall off. While I was paralysed with vertigo, I experienced my life as a juxtaposition of terrifying snapshots.'

That image clearly demonstrated that equilibrium results from the combination in space and time of various positions, each unstable by itself. Even if there is immobilization in a position of equilibrium, that immobilization is rarely passive but reflects the need to strike a balance between complementary forces. Those who have done isometric exercises know that well, and so do some psychoanalysts who discover that the way to sit up all day without getting a backache is to adopt an active sitting posture and not to sit slumped in a well-padded armchair.

The image of the swing did not satisfy Luc for long, his dissatisfaction proving that he was now in dynamic pursuit of equilibrium and no longer content to leave it at what he had already discovered; that image seemed too static for him: a swing executes a repetitive movement and has no real displacement in space. Luc then hit upon the image of a bicycle: to keep your balance on it you have to cycle ahead; should fear immobilize you, you fall off. But even that still seemed too linear an image to him; instead he imagined an aeroplane moving not only forward but upwards as well, or a swimmer freely parting the water. Yet even these images struck him as being too simple when compared with the complexity of life and with all the many factors we combine to create our present, which in turn modifies our past and prepares our future. How then are we to picture duration in that combination of time and space?

Between vertigo and equilibrium: playing with time

Freezing time or fitting a moment into time?

Freedom to play with time strikes me as being characteristic of the pursuit of equilibrium, while the tendency to freeze time would seem to accompany a leaning towards vertigo. I was quite familiar with Luc's attempts to stop time. Before the vacation, he would sometimes lie on the couch like a stone effigy. He did not budge, and the hands of the watch looked frozen to me. It was as if Luc had the magical power to stop time, as if the session would never end; in that way there would not only be no break for the vacation, there would never be any break at all, there would be no more death. By enacting death unconsciously, Luc could appear very powerful and deceive even death itself, but at the same time he seemed to have no life. With his omnipotent unconscious effort to freeze the moment, Luc was trying to ward off separation anxiety and the fear of death, but he ended up even more petrified with anxiety than he had been. In this wish to stop time we can sense how much vertigo and equilibrium are at the very heart of the interplay of the life and death drives.

As Luc described his first attack of vertigo on the girder, I could sense that the vertigo disappeared when time had resumed its advance; once the moment of victory could be related to the past and the future it became part of a history endowed with a wide range of meanings that spared Luc from vertigo. That is why I consider it so important to look closely at Luc's dissatisfaction: his images of a swing, of a bicycle and of a swimmer admittedly took account of space, of a displacement towards the future, but psychic balance is much more complex than that, and also implies playing with time.

In search of equilibrium: creating our own history

To convey a better idea of this creation based on the integration of the concept of time, I shall start with an example: a patient had ostensibly 'forgotten' an event in his life, had let it fall out of his personal history, rediscovered it during analysis, and then fitted it back into his conscious history. Here I do not wish to examine the details of this reconstruction, but simply to show how Serge was able to develop his picture of his personal history in the course of analysis, as he came to realize that his acts of forgetting were not the passive result of a constitutional shortcoming but the result of active psychic work on his part, naturally of an unconscious kind. It seemed obvious to me that the richer and more complex his imagery, the closer an analysand is to the register of psychic equilibrium and the further away he is from the register of vertigo.

Thirty years of forgetfulness

For thirty years Serge had forgotten his parents telling him that an important family member had died just before Serge was born. When he became aware of that act of forgetfulness during his analysis, the first idea to spring to his mind was that of a jigsaw puzzle one of whose pieces was missing. Until his analysis, the story of that death had remained an isolated moment of his childhood kept out of his consciousness. This severance of the links between that event and his own history was for Serge, rather as for Luc with his girder, a means of keeping perpetually alive while others died, and to keep out of one's conscious history all the anxieties such omnipotence entails: he had behaved as if the announcement of this relative's death could have no possible influence on his own life, so that there was no need to connect that event with his personal history. His spatial image of isolated jigsaw pieces corresponded, in its static character, to his temporal image of time cut up into isolated moments.

More generally, I have found that many analysands who complain of forgetting everything often have the static phantasy of being *sieves* or *riddles*, reified representations of their psyche considered as a passive container, a simple receptacle of juxtaposed, heterogeneous objects. These analysands do not see themselves in the process of creating a dynamic *system* of significations that would enable them to recover memories thanks to the meaningful place each of them occupies in the system as a whole. For lack of a link to the patient's psychic life at large, these moments become frozen into so many snapshots, and their meaning for the patient cannot develop as a function of the rest of his history.

Avoiding contamination by freezing time

By isolating in time a moment in their lives invested with too much anxiety, these analysands often try unconsciously to prevent their anxiety from contaminating their history, but at the same time prevent these anxious moments from being changed by other experiences that might have rendered them more tolerable. These patients who 'freeze time to kill the memory' (D. Quinodoz 1990a) give me the impression of eliciting vertigo while unconsciously believing that they are avoiding it.

In fact, when a frightening event is frozen out of the patient's lifetime, like a piece apart from the rest of the jigsaw puzzle, that event can weigh most heavily on the patient's life. The momentary event can assume the status of a timeless object, pressing down the more heavily on the patient's life the more it is excluded from the development of his internal objects, from his history, and not making its presence felt only through acting out. This confers a magical and dizzying omnipotence upon this isolated moment: thus Serge, who invariably had the impression that he was not wanted, felt that all his interlocutors were waiting for someone better and that they were disappointed to find Serge instead. It was as if he imagined unconsciously that his interlocutors were expecting someone who had died before his birth, and not him. This analysand had several episodes of expansion-related vertigo when he became aware of his own psychic structure, so much did he dread the sadness that went with the reunification of his ego.

In dealing with patients I have often been amazed to discover the importance in their lives of grave moments they were unable to turn into memories fitting into their history, for instance, the death of a parent which was kept from the child under the impression that it would be less painful for him were he to find out about it later. That event then lingers on like a inert mass in the patient's life, instead of developing along with the rest of his history. Now a person cannot be divorced from his history; if he attempts to do that, part of himself will seem devitalized. By contrast, when the patient is able to link an anxious moment to his internal objects, that moment will henceforth be constantly reshaped in keeping with the development of the patient's inner world; he sheds his omnipotence, and invests time with a wealth of subtle shades of meaning, enabling him to look at the moment from various angles that help to relativize it and hence to render it less fraught with anxiety.

The stability of immobile phenomena: an illusion

It proved a great shock for Serge to discover the relationship between time and anxiety during his analysis. He gradually found out that the stability of immobile phenomena was an illusion (the immobilization of the dead relative outside Serge's own history) and that it was, on the contrary, thanks to movement and time that he was able to find equilibrium, which had to be recreated all the time. His life then began to look to him like *a walk* – while we walk, we keep our balance thanks to a movement which, combining space and time, enables us to link positions each of which, taken in isolation, is unstable. Serge then went on to think of the work involved in linking up events in his life the better to fit them into a history, as a thread on which one can string pearls to fashion a necklace instead of leaving them scattered about at random.

However, this picture of a *thread linking the pearls* of his memory soon struck him as being too linear, as constituting a simple chronology rather than a process in time. And what disturbed him most in that picture of memories strung together like pearls was that the nature of the string joining them together was different from that of the pearls, whereas time is a movement constituting an integral part of the structure of every element, animating the whole at one stroke. The qualitative difference between the two may be likened to the difference between a *line* that a brilliant painter, filled with creative inspiration, might have drawn with a continuous stroke, and a *copy* of that line made by joining it together point by point.

His various ideas of time in its double – continuous and discontinuous –

aspect, together with the representations of the various possible articulations of the moments constituting continuous time, enabled Serge to construct a picture of the different ways in which he could compose his own history based on what he had experienced. Some moments of his life, split off from the rest, might appear as loose pearls devoid of significant context; other moments might seem like isolated pearls even though connected by the linear thread of the necklace; while the well-integrated moments of his history were like the *musical phrases* of a symphony, or perhaps like the *separate organs of one and the same constantly evolving body*. In the last two cases, the whole is made up of the combination of various parts, each of which owes its meaning to the presence of the whole. We can understand that at the end of his analysis, the picture of the missing jigsaw piece no longer satisfied Serge because it was much too static; it did not account for the inner movement which ensures that, at every moment, the self, fitting into the time constituting its history, modifies its past and lends it meaning, thus shaping the future.

It is sometimes by rediscovering in analysis the possibility of playing with time that a patient discovers a vital meaning in a past event, fits it into his history and so avoids what it might lead to in the form of vertiginous anxiety. We saw that this happened when Luc refitted the girder episode into his personal history; as a result that episode assumed a new and previously unknown significance and lost its ability to affect Luc's life without his knowledge. 'Two different analysands speaking about their past may say, "*that page has now been turned*", but for one it means "that page has been torn out, thrown into the waste-paper basket, don't let's talk about it any more", while for the other it means, "I have turned that page, true enough, but only after having read it"; this presupposes that what he has just read will influence his reading of the following pages, but also that his reading of the following pages will modify his understanding of the earlier pages of the book' (D. Quinodoz 1992a: 20).

Omnipotence or realistic power? Vertigo or disequilibrium? The ability to symbolize

At the end of his analysis, Luc was able, thanks to a dream, to come up with representations of the double attitude characteristic of patients suffering from vertigo: an infantile attitude trying for success in the register of omnipotence and a more highly developed attitude operating in the register of realistic power; the dream made it quite clear that these two attitudes are incompatible. What was so interesting in his report of that dream was that Luc realized that he himself was playing all the parts in that dream, which enabled him to adopt, at the level of phantasy, the most diverse attitudes.

Here then is the dream: Luc took part in a competition to establish who had the longest penis. The rules of the competition were that every penis had to be measured while it was flaccid. But one competitor cheated because he kept his penis permanently erect, and Luc identified with that cheat inasmuch as he too was mainly concerned to prove his omnipotence, even if that meant freezing time at the peak of this illusory victory; in short, he was one to whom the competition was not something to be judged by objective criteria. But Luc was also the judge: what was he to do? To disqualify the cheat or to punish him? The incompatibility of the two registers became obvious: as judge he could not allow a person vying for omnipotent victory to participate in a competition run in the register of realistic power. Moreover, the omnipotent victory was dangerous, because it might bring castration as a punishment.

This dream allowed Luc to get a picture of all the possibilities at war inside him during his attacks of vertigo. Moreover, in his dream and his phantasy he was allowing himself to satisfy previously unconscious wishes and also to face old problems he had since analysed and integrated. He appreciated the freedom enjoyed by the analysand who has discovered that having phantasies is not the same as acting them out.

I believe that a dream like that, at the end of an analysis, is one of those integrative dreams to which J.-M. Quinodoz has referred as 'page-turning dreams', that is, 'dreams in which an entire phantasised situation that he [the patient] has just abandoned appears with astonishing accuracy. . . . The dream then renders the phantasy content accessible, because in it "thing-presentations" meet "word-presentations"'(1987: 837). Reporting such dreams, by which the analysand arrives at representations, opens the way for symbolism. Now everything that can be symbolized seems to me to be snatched from the jaws of vertigo and moved closer to the equilibrium pole, affording the analysand a better integration of the infantile part of his ego.

Vertigo and equilibrium

The duality of extremes: the motor force of equilibrium

Vertigo and equilibrium lie at the crossroads of change and immutability. I have described different moments in the construction of relational space corresponding to various forms of vertigo and the pursuit of equilibrium; these creations of space range from the bi-dimensional world in which the void itself has no place, through the apprehension of the void, a negative space manifesting a denial of the absence of relations, to the construction of tri-dimensional space in which the analysand often gains the impression that he is being held up by the object before discovering that he can hold himself up, and finally to the construction of the internal space that permits the internalization of the feeling of buoyancy. The various forms of equilibrium do not exclude but complete one another and combine, interpenetrating, modifying and being modified in turn, like the movements of a symphony.

I believe that if we had to stress just one approach to the study of the anxiety presented by analysands who are torn between vertigo and equilibrium, we should be looking at the psychic process that has accompanied us throughout this book: that of analysands ceaselessly trying to contain and to combine extremes within themselves. These extremes may sometimes be irreconcilable, for instance when the analysand, in the grip of vertigo, must begin to close an internal split and, say, help his infantile part to develop before he can integrate it. There may also be reconcilable extremes, for instance when the analysand, having abandoned the register of vertigo for that of equilibrium, must combine reconcilable forces that, separately, would pull him in opposite directions. These extremes, which are so many forces present in the analysand, can be felt in an infinite range of the most diverse spheres.

The analysand can be thrown into great confusion when he senses the presence of these opposite forces in him but fails to see any possibility of combining them into a result. He gains greater equilibrium every time he tries in a creative way to combine two extreme tendencies in order to arrive at a synthesis; that is, whenever he joins two components into a whole that is greater than the components without destroying them; this process implies a qualitative difference between the result and its components. Throughout this book we have had occasion, during the discussion of the analysis of various patients, to look at the various spheres in which they may encounter and have to combine opposite aspirations: love and hate, fusion and differentiation, immobility and movement, permanence and transience, smallness and immensity, emptiness and fullness, internal and external – the list can grow very long indeed.

Everything in us develops and yet something immovable remains, be it only the paradoxical certainty that our identity persists throughout our life. That certainty is paradoxical because our appearance keeps changing as we progress from birth to maturity; how then is it that, from the baby weighing a few pounds to the old man or woman we may become, we have the feeling of always being the same person? It was this strange fact that made Luc exclaim at the end of his analysis: 'I keep developing and yet I remain myself; and the other always remains himself, even if he has changed and renewed almost every cell in his body.' In order not to suffer from vertigo during that ever-changing process, Luc felt the need to seek this 'stable' element in his own centre and said, 'Even the earth on which I stand keeps turning; I cannot rely on the outside but must seek my centre of gravity in myself.'

The different facets through which we may come to grips with the basic duality of our drives

Freud spoke of the duality of the life and death drives. I believe that every analyst comes up, in his clinical practice, against the conflicting drives present in every one of his patients, and that these conflicts create a basic dynamism, serve as an essential motor force, without which everything would grind to a halt. What we have here are not two external forces pulling the analysand in different directions, but internal forces, being part of the analysand himself, and needing his integrative action so that, instead of cancelling each other out and leading to immobility, they produce a result which acts as a motor force. It is in this sense, as Melanie Klein argued, that anxiety becomes a motor of psychic life.

In theory, it is quite possible to reduce these conflicts to a basic one, namely to a conflict between two drives encompassing all the other dualities. However, in analysis, patients and analyst are confronted with a variety of facets adopted, with the passage of time, by the extreme forms triggering off the analysand's vital movement. In effect, the drives cannot be grasped directly but must be apprehended through their psychic representatives and the affects accompanying them. The psychic representatives themselves assume quite distinct forms with every analysand, and there is an infinity of means of manifesting one's destructive and libidinal forces, every analysand creating his own way. What I find so fascinating in psychoanalysis is the discovery of the diversity with which analysands can experience the presence of extremes in them and try for equilibrium.

Some artists have been particularly good at expressing, in their work, the integration of extremes with its surprising and fragile aspects. I am thinking particularly of the work of the Swiss sculptor, Jean Tinguely. There is no need for long arguments to make it clear to one and all what equilibrium is: a precarious state, resulting from various movements and unstable positions, which a single speck of dust might upset. It is, in effect, the privilege of works of art to make us feel what is so difficult to explain in words. The integrative capacity of the human psyche can, of course, be described; we can make a list of the conditions needed if it is to function properly, in the same way that we can analyse the quality of the canvas and the composition of colours Rembrandt needed to create his *Night Watch*. However, what constitutes the very essence of the integration of beauty and psychic creation is something I do not believe we can explain properly. And that is all to the good: long may the human spirit keep surprising us.

Bibliography

Abraham, K. (1913) 'A constitutional basis of locomotor anxiety', in *Selected Papers on Psycho-Analysis*, London: Hogarth: 235–43.

Anouilh, J. (1951) *Antigone* (trans. Lewis Galantière), London: Methuen.

Anzieu, D. (1987) 'Les signifiants formels et le moi-peau', in *Les enveloppes psychiques*, Paris: Dunod: 1–22.

Balint, M. (1959) *Thrills and Regressions*, London: Hogarth.

Bick, E. (1968) 'The experience of the skin in early object relations', in *International Journal of Psycho-Analysis*, 49: 484––6.

Bion, W. R. (1962) *Learning from Experience*, London: Heinemann.

—— (1967) *Second Thoughts*, London: Karnac.

Chasseguet-Smirgel, J. (1964) 'La culpabilité féminine', in *Recherches psychiatriques nouvelles sur la sexualité féminine*, Paris: Presses universitaires de France: 129–80.

Degoumois, C. (1992) 'La nuit d'Icare, paradoxe du somnambule', lecture read to the Centre de Psychanalyse R. de Saussure, 14 November 1992, unpublished.

Diatkine, R. (1988) 'Destins du transfert', in *Revue française de psychanalyse*, 4: 803–12.

—— (1992) 'Le concept d'objet et l'analyse du transfert', in *Bulletin Fédération Européenne de Psychanalyse*, 39: 57–69.

Donnet, J. L. and Green, A. (1973) *L'enfant de ça. Psychanalyse d'un entretien: la psychose blanche*, Paris: Minuit.

Duperey, A. (1992) *Le voile noir*, Paris: Seuil.

Ferenczi, S. (1914), 'Sensations of giddiness at the end of the psycho–analytic session', in *Further Contributions to the Theory and Technique of Psycho-Analysis*, London: Hogarth (1926): 239–41.

French, T. M. (1929) 'Psychogenic material related to the function of the semi-circular canals', in *International Journal of Psycho-Analysis*, 10: 398–410.

The references to Freud's work have been arranged in accordance with the bibliographical references of the *Standard Edition of the Complete Psychological Works of Sigmund Freud*, 24 vols. London: Hogarth, 1953–73.

Freud, S. (1887–1902) *The Origins of Psycho-Analysis* (Letters to Wilhelm Fliess, Drafts and Notes), London: Imago (1954); included in S.E. 1: 175–397.

—— (1895b [1894]) 'On the grounds for detaching a particular syndrome from neurasthenia under the description of "anxiety neurosis"', S.E. 3: 87–117.

—— (1895d [1893—895]) *Studies on Hysteria*, S.E. 2.

—— (1900a) *The Interpretation of Dreams*, S.E. 4–5.

—— (1905d) *Three Essays on the Theory of Sexuality*, S.E. 7: 125–243.

—— (1909b) 'Analysis of a phobia in a five-year-old boy', S.E. 10: 3–149.

—— (1915c) 'Instincts and their vicissitudes', S.E. 14: 111–40.

—— (1916–1917) *Introductory Lectures on Psycho-Analysis*, S.E. 15-16.

—— (1917c) 'On transformations of instinct as exemplified in anal eroticism', S.E. 17: 127–33.

—— (1920) *Beyond the Pleasure Principle*, S.E. 20: 1–64.

—— (1922a) 'Dreams and telepathy', S.E. 18: 197–220.

—— (1923a [1922]) 'Two encyclopaedia articles', S.E. 18: 235–59.

—— (1923b) *The Ego and the Id*, S.E. 19: 3–66.

—— (1924c) 'The economic problem of masochism', S.E. 19: 157–70.

—— (1926d) *Inhibitions, Symptoms and Anxiety*, S.E. 20: 77–175.

—— (1930a) *Civilization and its Discontents*, S.E. 21: 59–145.

—— (1933a) *New Introductory Lectures on Psycho-analysis*, S.E. 22: 3–182.

—— (1940a [1938]) *An Outline of Psycho-Analysis*, S.E. 23: 141–207.

—— (1993) *Sigmund Freud and Sandor Ferenczi, The Correspondence of, 1908–1914*, vol. 1, Cambridge, Mass.: Harvard University Press.

Gibeault, A. (1989) 'Destins de la symbolisation', Rapport au XLIXe Congrès des Psychanalystes de Langue Française des Pays Romans, in *Revue française de psychanalyse*, 6: 1517–18.

Green, A. (1971) 'La projection: de l'identification projective au projet', in *La folie privée*, Paris: Gallimard (1990): 195–223.

—— (1980) 'Le silence du psychanalyste', in *Topique*, 23: 5–25.

—— (1983) *Narcissisme de vie, narcissisme de mort*, Paris: Éditions de Minuit.

Grinberg, L. (1985) *Teoria de la identificación*, Madrid: Tecnipublicaciones.

Haag, G. (1991a) 'De la sensorialité aux ébauches de pensée chez les enfants autistes', in *Revue internationale de psychopathologie*, 3: 51–63.

—— (1991b) 'Some reflections on body ego development through psychotherapeutic work with an infant', in *Extending Horizons* (eds R. Szur and S. Miller), London: Karnac.

Häusler, R. (1985) 'Vertiges et troubles d'équilibre', in *Journal: Questions et Réponses*, Basel: *Internationale Medizinische Publikationen*, 5: 5–25.

—— (1989) Duplicated lecture notes on vertigo, Faculty of Medicine, Geneva.

Hugo, V. (1838) *Ruy Blas*, Paris: Gallimard Nouvelle Revue Française (Ed. La Pléiade).

Jones, E. (1953) *The Life and Work of Sigmund Freud*, London: Hogarth.

Klein M. (1929) 'Infantile anxiety situations reflected in a work of art and in the creative impulse', in *The Writings of Melanie Klein I*, London: Hogarth (1975): 210–18.

—— (1932) *The Psycho-Analysis of Children*, London: Virago (1989).

—— (1934) 'A contribution to the psychogenesis of manic–depressive states', in *The Writings of Melanie Klein I*, London: Hogarth (1975): 262–89.

—— (1946) 'Notes on some schizoid mechanisms', in *Envy and Gratitude and Other Works 1946-1963*, London: Hogarth (1975): 1–24.

—— (1948) 'On the theory of anxiety and guilt', in *Envy and Gratitude and Other Works 1946–1963,* London: Hogarth (1975): 25–42.

—— (1957) 'Envy and gratitude', in *Envy and Gratitude and Other Works 1946–1963*, London: Hogarth (1975): 176–235.

—— (1963) 'On the sense of loneliness', in *Our Adult World and Other Essays*, London: Heinemann: 102–8.

Kundera, M. (1985) *The Unbearable Lightness of Being*, London: Faber.

Laplanche, J. and Pontalis, J.-B. (1967) *Vocabulaire de la psychanalyse*, Paris: Presses Universitaires de France.

—— (1988) *The Language of Psycho-Analysis* (trans. D. Nicholson-Smith), London: Karnac.

Leymarie J. (1984) *Van Gogh*, Geneva: Skira.

Mann, T. (1928) *The Magic Mountain* (trans. H. T. Lowe-Porter), Harmondsworth: Penguin, 19.

McDougall, J. (1964) 'Considérations sur la relation d'objet dans l'homosexualité féminine', in *Recherches psychanalytiques sur la sexualité féminine*, Paris: Payot: 221–74.

Meltzer, D. (1975) 'Adhesive identification', in *Contemporary Psycho-Analysis*, 2: 289–310.

—— (1984) 'Les concepts d "identification projective" (Klein) et de "contenant–contenu" (Bion), en relation avec la situation analytique', in *Revue française de psychanalyse*, 2: 541–50.

—— (1986) 'Le conflit esthétique', in *Bulletin du Groupe d'Études et de Recherches sur la Psychologie de l'Enfant et du Nourrisson*, 6: 1–15.

Messner, R. (1978) *Grenzbereich Todeszone*, Cologne: Kiepenheuer; quoted from the Italian translation, *Limite della vita* (1980), Bologna: Zanichelli.

—— (1980) *Solo Nanga Parbat* (trans. Audrey Salkeld), London: Kaye & Ward.

—— (1989) *Die schönsten Gipfel der Welt*, Künzelsau: Sigloch.

Montaigne, M. (1580) *Les Essais*, Paris: Garnier (1962).

Montandon, P. and Lehmann, W. (1992) *Cours d'oto-rhinolaryngologie et de chirurgie cervico-faciale*, Geneva: Médicine et Hygiène.

Pascal, B. (n.d.) *Pensées et opuscules*, Paris: L. Brunschwicg-Hachette.

Petit, P. (1991) *Funambule*, Paris: Albin Michel.

Pragier, G. and Faure-Pragier, S. (1990) 'Un siècle après l'*Esquisse*: nouvelles métaphores? Métaphores de nouveau', in *Revue française de psychanalyse*, 6: 1395–502.

Prévert, J. (1947) 'Le jardin', *Paroles*, in *Œuvres complètes*, Paris: NRF, La Pléiade (1949).

Quinodoz, D. (1984a) 'L'accident en tant que révélateur de la pulsion de mort', Symposium Fédération Européenne de Psychanalyse sur la pulsion de mort, Marseille (1984) in *Bulletin de la Société suisse de Psychanalyse*, 17: 4–8 and *Bulletin Fédération Européenne de Psychanalyse* (1985), 25: 95–9.

—— (1984b) 'L'incapacité de bien traiter ses objects internes comme expression de l'homosexualité latente', in *Revue française de psychanalyse*, 3: 745–50.

—— (1986) 'Don Juan, serait-il hystérique?', in *Revue française de psychanalyse*, 3: 1005–8.

—— (1987) '"J'ai peur de tuer mon enfant" ou Œdipe abandonné, Œdipe adopté', in *Revue française de psychanalyse*, 6: 1579–93; 'Ich habe Angst mein Kind zu töten', in *Zeitschrift für psy. Theorie und Praxis* (1991) 1: 47–61.

—— (1989a) 'L'objet serait-il avant tout corporel?', in *Revue française de psychanalyse*, 4: 1142–4.

—— (1989b) 'Le symbolon: gage de lien ou de rupture?', in *Revue française de psychanalyse*, 6: 1648–52.

—— (1990a) 'Figer le temps pour tuer le souvenir' in *Revue française de psychanalyse*, 4: 1001–6.

—— (1990b) 'L'insoutenable incertitude: le fantasme du berceau vide', in *Revue française de psychanalyse*, 6: 1567–72.

—— (1990c) 'Vertigo and object relationship', in *International Journal of Psycho-Analysis*, 71: 53–63.

—— (1991a) 'Vieillir: appauvrissement ou enrichissement?', in *Psychothérapies*, 1: 27–32.

—— (1991b) 'À la recherche du sujet perdu', in *Revue française de psychanalyse*, 6: 1689–95.

—— (1992a) 'La construction du souvenir', in *Bulletin de la Société Suisse de Psychanalyse*, 34: 18–20.

—— (1992b) 'The psychoanalytical setting as the instrument of the container function' in *International Journal of Psycho-Analysis*, 73: 627–36.

—— (1994) 'Interpretations in projection', *International Journal of Psychoanalysis*, 75: 755–61.

—— (1996) 'An adopted analysand's trahsference of a "hole-object"', *International Journal of Psycho-Analysis*, 77: 323–36.

Quinodoz, J.-M. (1987) 'Des "rêves qui tournent la page"', in *Revue française de psychanalyse*, 2: 837–8.

—— (1991b) 'Accepter la fusion pour en sortir', in *Revue française de psychanalyse*, 6: 1697–700.

Quinodoz, J.-M. (1993) *The Taming of Solitude* (trans. Philip Slotkin), London: Routledge.

Rank, O. (1924) *Das Trauma der Geburt* (English translation: *The Trauma of Birth* (1929)), London: Kegan Paul.

Rallo, J. (1972) 'Aggressiveness, feelings of giddiness and muscular tension,' in *International Journal of Psycho-Analysis*, 53: 265–9.

Rentchnick, P. and Häusler, R. (1985) 'Dialogues thérapeutiques', in *Médecine et Hygiène*, 1627: 3096–8.

Rycroft, C. (1953) 'Some observations on a case of vertigo', in *International Journal of Psycho-Analysis*, 341: 241–7.

Schilder, P. (1939) 'The relation between clinging and equilibrium', in *International Journal of Psycho-Analysis*, 20: 58–63.

Schur, M. (1972) *Freud: Living and Dying*, New York: International Universities Press.

Segal, H. (1957) 'Notes on symbol formation', in *The Work of Hanna Segal*, London: Free Association Books and Maresfield Reprints (1986): 49–68.

—— (1973) *Introduction to the Work of Melanie Klein*, London: Karnac (1988).

—— (1979) *Klein*, London: Fontana.

—— (1990) 'What is an object? The role of perception', in European Psycho-analytical Federation, *Bulletin* 35.

Skopek, L. and Carreras, R. (1988), *S'envoler sans s'affoler*, Geneva: Sécavia.

Spira, M. (1985) *Créativité et liberté psychique*, Lyon: Césura.

Spitz, R.A. (1953) *La première année de la vie de l'enfant*, Paris: Presses Universitaires de France.

Staël, N. de (1981) *Lettres à Jacques Dubourg*, London: Taranman (no page numbers).

Van Gogh, V. (1958) *The Complete Letters of Vincent van Gogh* (ed. and trans. Johanna van Gogh-Bonner), London: Thames and Hudson.

—— (1990) *De brieven van Vincent van Gogh*, The Hague: SDU Uitgeverij.

—— (1996) *The Letters of Vincent van Gogh* (ed. Ronald de Leeuw and trans. Arnold Pomerans), London: Allen Lane.

Name Index

Subject Index

Printed in the United States
by Baker & Taylor Publisher Services

Printed in the United States
by Baker & Taylor Publisher Services